Respiratory Physiology
in Anesthetic Practice

Respiratory Physiology in Anesthetic Practice

THOMAS J. GAL, M.D.

Professor of Anesthesiology
University of Virginia Health Sciences Center
Charlottesville, Virginia

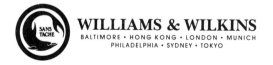

WILLIAMS & WILKINS
BALTIMORE · HONG KONG · LONDON · MUNICH
PHILADELPHIA · SYDNEY · TOKYO

Editor: Timothy H. Grayson
Associate Editor: Linda Napora
Copy Editor: Thomas Lehr
Designer: Norman W. Och
Illustration Planner: Lorraine Wrzosek
Production Coordinator: Raymond E. Reter

Accurate indications, adverse reactions, and dosage schedules for drugs are provided in this book, but it is possible that they may change. The reader is urged to review the package information data of the manufacturers of the medications mentioned.

Printed in the United States of America

Library of Congress Cataloging-in-Publication Data

Gal, Thomas J.
    Respiratory physiology in anesthetic practice / Thomas J. Gal.
      p. cm.
    Includes bibliographical references and index.
    ISBN 0-683-03414-6
    1. Anesthetics—Physiological effect.   2. Respiratory organs—
Effect of drugs on.   3. Respiration—Regulation.   4. Respirators.
I. Title.
    [DNLM: 1. Anesthesia.   2. Respiration—drug effects.
3. Respiration—physiology.   4. Respiration, Artificial.   WO 200
G146r]
RD82.G35   1992
617.9′6—dc20
DNLM/DLC
for Library of Congress   91-7399
                                      CIP
                                      Rev.

91 92 93 94 95
1 2 3 4 5 6 7 8 9 10

Preface

The clinical practice of anesthesiology demands a considerable knowledge of respiratory physiology. Current texts on the subject are either very lengthy and extensive or not directly related to anesthesiology. As a single-author text, this book is not intended to provide authoritarian information on a broad and comprehensive scale, nor is it intended to serve as an introductory text or handbook. Rather, the purpose is to provide the clinician with a concise base of information in a limited range of topics, all of which are relevant to the everyday practice of anesthesiology. These topics include respiratory mechanics, control of respiration, pulmonary circulation, gas exchange, and the physiology of mechanical ventilation.

The material is presented as a series of discussions, the content of which was stimulated by questions posed to me by residents, colleagues, and practitioners over the years. The information is not presented in a format that deals in minute detail with the management of specific conditions, equipment, or disease states, as might be found in handbooks. Instead there is a review of current concepts in respiratory physiology, which hopefully will enrich the clinician's perspective.

Assembly of the material for this book was indeed an enjoyable experience. During this endeavor I was encouraged by the continuous stream of questions posed by colleagues. The questions invariably related to topics dealt with in the text. For such encouragements, which indirectly contributed to the contents of the book, I must thank my fellow anesthesiologists at the University of Virginia. However, my deepest gratitude must be reserved for my loving wife, Mary Jane, who endured life with me during the preparation of the book. More importantly, her superb typing skills and capable editorial assistance made preparation of the text remarkably efficient and smooth.

Contents

vii

V APPENDICES

Respiratory Mechanics: The Respiratory System as an Air Pump

Chapter 1

Basic Mechanics of the Respiratory System

Any understanding of respiratory physiology must begin with a consideration of respiratory mechanics. This area of physiology deals with the role of the respiratory system as an air pump. It involves the analysis of the forces responsible for the physical transport of air into and out of the gas exchange portion of the system, i.e.,the lung. These forces act against other elements that oppose the airflow.

RESPIRATORY MUSCLES: THE FORCE GENERATORS

Air moves into and out of the lungs as the thoracic cavity expands and contracts, increasing and decreasing in size. This volume change is accomplished by the contraction and relaxation of the respiratory muscles. Functionally these are skeletal muscles whose primary task is to displace the chest wall rhythmically. There are three major muscle groups responsible for ventilation: the diaphragm, the intercostal muscles, and the accessory muscles. Although the functions of these muscles will be considered individually, it is most important to remember that they actually must work together in a coordinated fashion.[1]

Diaphragm

The diaphragm is a dome-shaped muscle that separates the thoracic cavity from the abdomen. The muscle is unique in that its fibers radiate from a central tendon to insert peripherally on the anterolateral aspects of the upper lumbar vertebrae (crural portion) and on the xiphoid and upper margins of the lower ribs (costal portion). The motor innervation originates from the phrenic nerve, which is formed by the combination of cervical roots 3, 4, and 5. Contraction of the diaphragm causes its dome to descend, thereby expanding the chest longitudinally. The attachments to costal margins also cause the lower ribs to rise and the chest to widen (Fig. 1.1). This action of the diaphragm is responsible

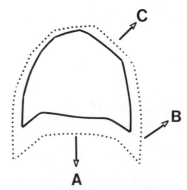

Figure 1.1. Diagrammatic representation of the thorax showing expansion from end expiration *(solid lines)* to end inspiration *(dotted lines)*. *A*, descent of diaphragm; *B*, lateral displacement due to diaphragmatic action on lower ribs and "bucket handle" motion of external intercostals; *C*, "pump handle" action of intercostals to elevate upper ribs and increase AP diameter.

for about two-thirds of quiet resting ventilation. The normal excursion of the diaphragm during such quiet breathing is about 1.5 cm. As the dome ascends to expand the thorax, the abdominal contents are displaced caudally. Thus the fall in pleural pressure and accompanying lung expansion produces an increase in abdominal pressure and some protrusion of the abdominal wall.

Intercostal Muscles

The intercostal muscles are composed of two sheet-like layers that run between the ribs; they receive their innervation from nerves that exit from the spinal cord at levels from the first to eleventh thoracic segments. The external intercostals and the parasternal portion of the internal intercostals produce an inspiratory action. Their contraction elevates the upper ribs to increase the anteroposterior dimensions of the chest (pump handle motion). The lower ribs are also raised to increase the transverse diameter of the thorax (bucket handle motion). Although these actions of the intercostals do not play a major role in normal resting ventilation, they are important in maintaining high levels of ventilation such as those required by exercise.

Accessory Muscles

The accessory muscles contribute to inspiration by elevating and stabilizing the rib cage. The principal accessory muscles are the scalenes and sternocleidomastoids. The scalenes originate from the transverse processes of the lower five cervical vertebrae and receive innervation from the same spinal segments. The muscles slope caudally to insert on the first two ribs so that contraction elevates and fixes the rib cage. While this plays only a minor role in quiet breathing, the enlargement of the upper chest is important at high levels of ventilation. The second group of accessory muscles, the sternocleidomastoids, elevate the sternum and increase the longitudinal dimensions of the thorax. They are also active only at high levels of ventilation and assume great importance in disease states associated with severe airway obstruction.

Expiratory Muscles

In contrast to the active phase of inspiration, expiration is passive during quiet breathing and occurs because of the elastic recoil of the respiratory system. However, when high levels of ventilation are required or if air movement is impeded by airway obstruction, expiration must involve active muscle contraction. This is achieved in part by the internal intercostal muscles which depress the ribs, but the major participants in active expiration are the abdominal muscles. These muscles, which form the ventrolateral abdominal wall, are innervated by the lower six thoracic and first lumbar nerves. They consist of the midline rectus abdominis and the internal and external oblique and transversus abdominis muscles laterally. These muscles act to displace the rib cage by pulling the lower ribs downward and inward. They also pull the abdominal wall inward and thus increase intraabdominal pressure. This displaces the diaphragm cranially into the thorax with a resultant increase in pleural pressure and decrease in lung volume at end expiration. In addition to their role as powerful muscles of expiration, the abdominal muscles are also important contributors to other respiratory activities, such as forced expiration and coughing and the nonrespiratory functions of defecation and parturition.

STATIC LUNG VOLUMES: DIMENSIONS OF THE RESPIRATORY SYSTEM

Definitions

To study the behavior of the respiratory system, it is useful to define its various dimensions. These are the subdivisions of gas volumes contained within the lungs during various breathing maneuvers. Although he was not the first to measure ventilatory volume,[2] John Hutchinson is credited with inventing the spirometer, coining the term vital capacity, and defining the functional subdivisions of lung volume.[3] The four major subdivisions of lung volume are residual volume (RV), tidal volume (VT), expiratory reserve volume (ERV), and inspiratory reserve volume (IRV). These four volumes can in turn be combined to form four capacities: total lung capacity (TLC), vital capacity (VC), inspiratory capacity (IC), and functional residual capacity (FRC). The relationships between these various lung volumes and capacities are illustrated in Figure 1.2 and defined in Table 1.1.

Measurements

Vital capacity and any of its components (VC, VT, ERV, IRV, and IC) can be measured with spirometry. The other three volumes (RV, FRC, and TLC) all

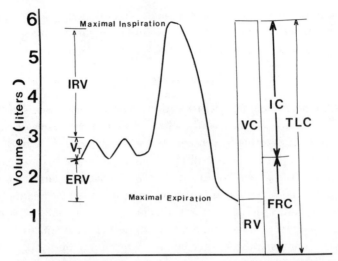

Figure 1.2. Volumes and capacities that make up the subdivisions of lung volume. Definitions and abbreviations are found in Table 1.1.

contain the residual volume (RV), which represents air not expressed from the lungs. Such a volume, therefore, must be measured by an indirect technique. In practice FRC is determined and RV calculated by subtracting the spirometrically obtained ERV from the measured FRC. Similarly, TLC can be calculated by adding the spirometric IC to FRC. This sequence is used because the resting end-expiratory level (FRC) is more easily maintained than a forced expiratory level (RV) or a maximal inspiratory level (TLC). Thus, measuring the more reproducible FRC ensures more consistent results in estimating lung volume.

Lung volume may be estimated from chest x-rays.[4] This is particularly true for TLC, which is the lung volume at which radiographs are usually taken. These techniques are somewhat less accurate than the more commonly used

Table 1.1.
Subdivisions of Static Lung Volumes

Tidal volume (V_T)—Volume of air inspired and expired with a quiet breath.
Residual volume (RV)—Volume of air in the lungs after a maximal expiration.
Expiratory reserve volume (ERV)—The volume of air that can be exhaled between the resting end-tidal position and RV.
Inspiratory reserve volume (IRV)—The volume of air inspired between the resting end-inspiratory position and a maximal inspiration.
Vital capacity (VC)—The amount of air expired from the point of maximal inspiration to the point of maximal expiration.
Total lung capacity (TLC)—Total volume of air in the lungs after a maximal inspiration. It is the sum of all subdivisions of lung volume.
Functional residual capacity (FRC)—Amount of air in the lungs at the end-tidal position. It is the sum of RV + ERV.

indirect techniques, which are two gas dilution methods (closed-circuit helium dilution and open-circuit nitrogen washout) and body plethysmography.

Closed-Circuit Helium Dilution

This technique is so named because the patient breathes while connected to a closed circuit that consists of either a bag of known volume or a spirometer containing a known concentration of helium. There is in turn no helium in the unknown volume of the patient's lungs at end expiration (FRC). The helium concentration is monitored while the rebreathing procedure continues for several minutes until the concentration of helium reaches equilibrium. Since no helium is absorbed or excreted while CO_2 absorption and O_2 addition keep the circuit volume relatively constant, FRC can be calculated:

$$\text{Initial system} \hspace{3cm} \text{Final system}$$
$$(\text{He concentration}) \times (\text{volume}) = (\text{He concentration}) \times (\text{volume})$$

Initial system volume is the known volume of the spirometer or bag, while the final system volume is this initial volume plus the patient's FRC. The latter is the only unknown in the equation.

Open-Circuit Nitrogen Washout

This techique is referred to as an open circuit because the patient breathes in from a source of 100% O_2 and exhales into a second circuit (bag or spirometer) that collects all of the expired gas. The measurement takes advantage of the fact that the N_2 concentration in the patient's lungs at the beginning is known (80%). As the patient continues to breathe 100% O_2, all the N_2 is washed out of the lungs and into the spirometer. This N_2 concentration can be measured with a nitrogen analyzer and the total expired volume determined with the spirometer.

$$(N_2 \text{ concentration}) \times (\text{gas volume}) = (N_2 \text{ concentration}) \times (\text{volume})$$
$$\text{Lungs} \hspace{4cm} \text{Expired gas}$$

Since the test begins at the end of a quiet expiration, the volume of gas in the lungs is the FRC and its N_2 concentration is assumed to be 80%.

Body Plethysmography

Functional residual capacity can also be determined by plethysmography, which is technically more complex but considered more accurate for measuring absolute lung volume.[5] The variable-pressure, constant-volume plethysmograph uses Boyle's law, which states that the product of alveolar pressure times lung volume is constant provided the temperature does not change. The subject sits inside a large airtight chamber and breathes quietly through a mouthpiece while a nose clip eliminates nasal breathing. A shutter closes at end exhalation and the subject is asked to pant lightly. The panting alternately compresses and expands the thorax as two transducers measure mouth and box pressures, which are plotted on an oscilloscope. Since no flow occurs, mouth pressure is assumed to be equal to alveolar pressure. Boyle's law can then be used to calculate the lung volume.

$$PV = (P + \Delta P)(V + \Delta V)$$

 P = alveolar pressure at end expiration (atmospheric pressure);
 V = volume of gas at end expiration (FRC);
ΔP = change in alveolar pressure sensed as changes in mouth pressure during panting efforts;
ΔV = change in gas volume during panting efforts, sensed as a change in box pressure.

Solving for V,

$$V = \Delta V/\Delta P \times (P + \Delta P)$$

Since P is small and can be disregarded,

$$V = P \text{ (barometric)} \times (\Delta V/\Delta P)$$

$\Delta V/\Delta P$ is the slope of the plot of box pressure versus mouth pressure on the oscilloscope. This depends on the volume of gas in the lungs when the shutter closes. The latter is usually FRC.

This technique is far faster than the dilution or washout techiques and allows several determinations to be obtained per minute. Perhaps the major disadvantage is the relatively high cost of the equipment required. In addition, some patients may be unable to enter the plethysmograph because of claustrophobia, skeletal abnormalities, or massive obesity.

Comparative Differences in Measurement of Lung Volume

In healthy subjects the volumes measured are comparable for all the techniques discussed. In patients with pulmonary disease significant differences may result. Body plethysmography measures the total intrathoracic volume that is compressed during panting. Gas dilution techniques measure only the volume of gas that communicates with the airways. In patients with obstructive airway disease some areas of the lung communicate poorly or not at all with the gas in the central airways. As a result, a significant underestimation of lung volume is possible with gas dilution techniques. Conversely, in patients with severe airway obstruction, plethysmographic estimates of lung volume may be falsely increased. This is most likely the result of differences between mouth and alveolar pressure as the relatively compliant upper airways narrow during rapid panting maneuvers. To minimize errors, patients with obstructive airway disease must be instructed to pant slowly (at a frequency less than 1 Hz) with good support of the cheeks to allow complete transmission of alveolar pressure to the mouth.[6]

Physiological Determinants of Lung Volume

A young adult male of average height would be likely to have a TLC of about 6.5 liters, of which 1.5 liters is residual volume. Therefore, vital capacity is about 5 liters. Differences in lung volumes among individuals are largely a function of differences in body size, in particular height. Other determinants of TLC include the strength of the inspiratory muscles and the elastic recoil properties of the lung and chest wall. The magnitude of RV is influenced primarily by expiratory muscle strength and the outward recoil of the chest wall. The limits of expiration may also be affected by dynamic airway closure, particularly with advancing age.[7] The volume at the end of a spontaneous exhalation during quiet breathing (FRC) corresponds to the resting volume of the respiratory system. At this volume airway pressure is zero, a reflection of the balance between the opposing recoil characteristics of the lung and chest wall.

The respiratory system and its component lung and chest wall are elastic. That is, they tend to regain their original size and configuration following deformation when deforming forces are removed. Both lung and chest wall have positions of equilibrium. These are the volumes that they tend to assume in the absence of external forces acting upon them, and the volumes to which they continuously attempt to return when displaced. The equilibrium position of the lung is at or near RV (Fig. 1.3**A**). To sustain any volume in the lung above RV, force must be applied to the lung and the lung will recoil with an equal and opposite force. At all volumes above RV, the lung recoils inward. The equilibrium position of the chest wall is at a relatively large volume, about 60% of vital capacity (Fig. 1.3**B**). To sustain any volume in the chest wall above this point, the chest wall must be actively enlarged by inspiratory muscle contraction, and it will tend to recoil inward in concert with the lung.

In the intact respiratory system, the lung and chest wall are coupled and work together. Behavior of the respiratory system is determined by the individual properties of the lung and chest wall. The equilibrium position of the respiratory system will be at the volume where the tendency of the lung to recoil inward is balanced by the tendency of the chest wall to recoil outward (Fig. 1.3). To sustain any volume in the respiratory system other than this resting volume, a force must be applied to displace both lung and chest wall. The recoil pressure of the respiratory system (Prs) that develops is the algebraic sum of the individual recoil pressures of the lung (PL) and the chest wall (Pcw).

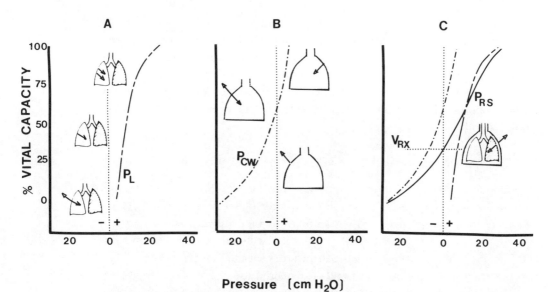

Pressure (cm H$_2$O)

Figure 1.3.   Pressure-volume relationships of the isolated lung (**A**), chest wall (**B**), and total respiratory system (**C**). Vrx, relaxation volume of the respiratory system (i.e., the resting equilibrium volume); PL, recoil pressure for the lung; Pcw, recoil pressure of the chest wall; Prs, recoil pressure for the total respiratory system.

Thus Prs = PL + Pcw. The volume at which Prs is zero is termed the resting or relaxation volume (Vrx) of the respiratory system. In normal persons during quiet breathing the volume of the lung at end expiration (FRC) approximates this Vrx. Under certain circumstances, however, FRC may differ from Vrx. Static factors such as respiratory muscle tone, posture, and external forces may reduce end-expiratory lung volume, while dynamic mechanisms may increase it.

The role of the elastic properties of the lung and chest wall and the relaxation pressure-volume characteristics of the respiratory system were delineated by having subjects relax their respiratory muscles as completely as possible as their airways were occluded at different lung volumes.[8] The pressures measured during these maneuvers reflect the elastic properties of the respiratory muscles of the rib cage. The extent to which respiratory muscle activity contributes to the relaxation pressures is difficult to assess. However, partial neuromuscular blockade by pancuronium produced a 15% decrease in FRC in six awake seated subjects.[9] The pressure-volume curve of the relaxed chest wall was shifted to the right so that its recoil or outward pull was decreased. Since lung recoil did not change, Vrx or FRC was decreased. In supine subjects partial paralysis did not affect FRC.[10] The latter observation suggests that the role of the respiratory muscles of the rib cage is less important in the supine posture.

Postural alterations in the pressure-volume relationships of the respiratory system are largely accounted for by the influence of gravity on the abdomen, which behaves mechanically like a fluid-filled container. In the erect posture the downward pull of gravity on the abdominal contents exerts an inspiratory action on the lungs by way of the diaphragm. In contrast, the action on the rib cage is more expiratory in nature. In the supine posture gravity also exerts a small expiratory action on the rib cage by pulling the ribs down and in but has a marked expiratory action on the diaphragm and abdomen. The pressure-volume curve for the chest wall is thus shifted to the right, i.e., it produces less opposition to the inward recoil of the lung. As a result, FRC in normals decreases from about 50% to about 40% TLC in the supine position, and even further to about 30% of TLC in the Trendelenburg position.[11] Interestingly, these striking changes with posture do not appear to be manifested in patients with pulmonary emphysema. The enlarged volumes for FRC in the latter are relatively less affected by body position.[12]

The static pressure-volume characteristics of the chest wall can be altered by externally applied forces. Restriction of the chest wall by strapping the rib cage or abdomen produces a marked decrease in FRC, primarily by limiting the tendency of the chest wall to recoil outward.[13] A somewhat similar displacement of the chest wall occurs in the seated subject submerged to the xiphoid or shoulder, much like the patient for shock wave lithotripsy. There is a decrease in FRC that is dependent on the depth of immersion.[14] Most of the decrease in lung volume reflects the inward displacement of the abdominal contents by the high hydrostatic pressure. The same hydrostatic pressure acting on the extremities may displace blood from the periphery to the lung and also contribute to the reduction in FRC.

Adult humans and most of the larger terrestrial mammals with relatively stiff chest walls breathe near their Vrx, and FRC is approximately equal to Vrx or about 50% TLC. The single exception to this is the horse, which appears to breathe around its Vrx with active inspiratory and expiratory phases so that FRC is less than Vrx. This respiratory pattern is believed to minimize the high elastic work of breathing,[15] since the latter is lowest when tidal volume is equally divided above and below Vrx.

During quiet breathing, there is ample time for emptying of the lungs to occur. If, however, ventilation must be increased (as, for example, during exercise) or emptying is delayed because of obstruction to flow, the end-expiratory lung volume may be determined by a dynamic rather than a static equilibrium. In obstructive lung disease, for example, FRC is commonly increased. Although an increase in resting lung volume (Vrx) may result from decreased lung elastic recoil, factors such as expiratory flow limitation may result in an even higher dynamically determined FRC.

The human newborn provides a particularly important example of a dynamically determined end-expiratory lung volume. The chest wall in infants and neonates is highly compliant, i.e., its outward recoil is exceedingly small. Although the inward recoil of the lungs is slightly less than in the adult, the lungs are relatively stiff compared to the chest wall. The static balance of elastic forces would predict an FRC at a very low lung volume (as low as 10% of TLC).[16] Since such a low lung volume seems incompatible with airway stability and adequate gas exchange, there is reason to suspect that the infant's dynamically determined FRC is substantially above the passive static Vrx. Olinsky et al. observed that in neonates the lung volume during apnea was lower than the usual end-expiratory level.[17]

Dynamic FRC is determined by the balance between two factors. The time available for expiration (TE) and the rate of lung emptying. The expiratory time (TE) is highly influenced by respiratory rates. In the neonate the rapid breathing frequency results in a relatively short TE. The rate of lung emptying is governed by the expiratory time constant (τ), which is essentially the product of resistance (R) and compliance (C). Because of the small size of the airways, neonates have an increased R and, because of the mechanical properties of the rib cage, a highly compliant chest wall (increased C). Thus τ, which equals R $\times$ C, is relatively prolonged. Whenever the ratio TE/τ is less than 3, dynamic FRC exceeds Vrx and airway pressure at end expiration does not reach zero. Such appears to be the case in the human neonate. The transition from this dynamically maintained FRC appears to occur at about 1 year of age.[18] At this point the end-expiratory level approximates Vrx, presumably because of changes in the mechanical properties of the lungs and chest wall as well as increases in TE.

FORCES INVOLVED IN BREATHING

Production of Airflow

Air flows in and out of the respiratory system because of differences in pressure. Flow occurs from a region of higher pressure to one of lower pressure. Basically, there are two pressure differences in the lung and another across the chest wall. The force driving airflow is the pressure differential between the airway opening or mouth (Pm) and the pressure in the alveoli (PA). This is termed the transairway pressure (Fig. 1.4**A**). The lung distends and collapses because of a pressure gradient between the alveoli (PA) and the pleural space (Ppl). This difference is termed transpulmonary pressure (PL), i.e., the pressure across the lung (Fig. 1.4**B**). The pressure across the chest wall (Pcw) (Fig. 1.4**C**) is reflected by the difference between the pleural pressure (Ppl) and the atmospheric or body surface pressure (Pbs).

Forces Opposing Airflow

Within the respiratory system certain elements oppose airflow and thus result in pressure drops. These forces opposing airflow are those resulting from the elastic, flow resistive, and inertial properties of the respiratory system. They are thus termed elastance, resistance, and inertance. Inertance deals with the mass of the lung and the acceleration of these tissues and the linear acceleration of gas in the lung. It is analogous to inductance in an electrical circuit.

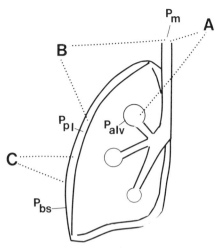

Figure 1.4.   Respiratory pressures at four sites: mouth (Pm), alveoli (Palv), pleural space (Ppl), and body surface (Pbs). *A*, transairway pressure (Palv − Pm; *B*, transpulmonary pressure (PL), the pressure across the lung (Palv − Ppl); *C*, pressure across the chest wall (Pcw) i.e., transthoracic pressure (Ppl − Pbs).

Thus, pressure losses due to inertial forces increase progressively as respiratory frequency increases. These pressure losses are quite small and negligible during quiet breathing and in most clinical situations. However, inertance may assume some importance during very rapid breathing, such as during exercise and other physiological testing. Elastance and its reciprocal, compliance, are reflections of the relationships of pressure to volume when there is no airflow. Hence such measurements are referred to as static. Resistance, on the other hand, is highly dependent on the rate of change of lung volume, i.e., flow. Such measurements during active breathing are referred to as dynamic.

Statics

The lung is a distensible elastic body enclosed in an elastic container, the thoracic cavity. Just as a spring is described by the force required to stretch it to a certain length, so can the respiratory system be described by the static pressure required to change its volume. This relation between changes in volume and changes in pressure is termed compliance ($\Delta V / \Delta P$), the reciprocal of elastance. For the various components of the respiratory system, compliance is determined by relating the change in volume to given pressure differences. These various pressures, as illustrated in Figure 1.4, are:

1. *Transpulmonary Pressure (PL) or Pressure across Lung:*
   PL = PA − Ppl
   PA = alveolar pressure. It is the same as mouth pressure (Pm) under condition of zero flow.
   Ppl = pleural pressure (usually sensed as esophageal pressure)

2. *Pressure across Chest Wall (Pcw):*
   Pcw = Ppl − Pbs
   Pbs = Pressure at body surface (atmospheric)
3. *Transrespiratory Pressure across Respiratory System (Prs)*
   Prs = PA − Pbs

Because the pressure-volume curves for the respiratory system are curvilinear (Fig. 1.3), compliance will vary from one portion of the curve to another depending on the range of lung volume. Values, therefore, are usually obtained in the range of 1 liter above FRC, where the pressure-volume relationships are most linear.

For many years, Ppl was estimated by using a special thin-walled balloon in the midesophagus. The balloon was 10 cm long and usually filled with 0.5 ml of air.[19] More recently, a 127-cm long nasogastric tube incorporating a similar balloon has become available commercially and has made the measurement more accessible to the clinician.[20] The pressure across the lung (PL) is thus measured by connecting the balloon to one port of a differential pressure transducer while the other port of the transducer senses mouth pressure.

It is important to make the distinction between the terms static and dynamic compliance. When no gas flow occurs and pressure and volume are kept constant, the measurement is termed static compliance. Such would be the case if the patient's lung were inflated by a device, such as a super syringe, and then held. Dynamic compliance, on the other hand, relates pressure and tidal volume at the moment inspiration changes to expiration and flow ceases only momentarily. Ideally, these two compliance measurements are similar. However, if flow is impeded for some reason, for instance by bronchoconstriction or a kink in the endotracheal tube, dynamic compliance is influenced by resistance to flow and does not reflect the true static compliance. They differ by an amount related to flow resistance at end inspiration. The difference between the peak dynamic pressures and a quasi-static pressure (plateau) can be readily appreciated in circuits utilizing a ventilator equipped with an inspiratory hold or pause, or by interrupting flow by merely clamping the expiratory tubing (Fig. 1.5). The relationship between delivered volume and the plateau pressure during this pause is often referred to as the "quasi-static" or "effective" compliance, while dynamic compliance relates to the relationship between delivered volume and peak dynamic pressure.

There is one final area of respiratory statics that deserves special comment. This concerns the relationship of the pressure in the alveoli (PA) in relation to alveolar size. According to Laplace's equation, the pressure within an alveolus (P) should exceed ambient pressure by an amount determined by the surface tension (T) and the radius of curvature (r) of the alveolus. Thus $P = 2T/r$. According to the equation, the pressure inside small alveoli should exceed that in larger ones if surface tension were the same. Thus one might expect the

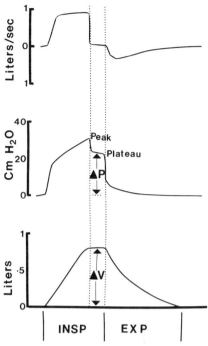

Figure 1.5. Diagrammatic representation of flow ($\dot{V}$), pressure (P), and tidal volume (VT) typical of a cycle of mechanical ventilation incorporating an inspiratory pause (area enclosed between *dotted lines*). (Reproduced with permission from Gal TJ. Monitoring the function of the respiratory system. In: Lake CL, ed. Clinical monitoring. 1st ed. Philadelphia: WB Saunders, 1989, Chapter 9.)

small alveoli to empty into larger ones. This problem is resolved by the fact that the surface tension of the fluid linking alveoli varies, decreasing as an alveolus decreases in size. The surface tension decreases to a greater extent than alveolar size (r). Therefore, the recoil pressure (P) of the small alveolus is less than that of the large ones. The lipoprotein substance responsible for this reduction of alveolar surface tension (surfactant) is secreted by type II pneumocytes and floats on the surface of the alveolar lining. As the lining surface decreases in area, surfactant concentration in the area increases and functions to decrease the surface tension of the lining fluid.

Dynamics

This deals with conditions of airflow and describes the relationships between pressure and flow in the respiratory system. Resistance therefore is computed from pressure differences responsible for flow and the simultaneous measurement of airflow ($R = \Delta P/\Delta \dot{V}$).

Various components of the respiratory system contribute to the total resistance to airflow. These include an elastic component, the chest wall, and a nonelastic component termed pulmonary resistance. Approximately 40% of total respiratory resistance is accounted for by the chest wall. It is important to note that the "chest wall" in physiologic terms includes not only the bony thorax but the diaphragm and abdominal contents as well. Therefore, changes in muscle tone may affect measurements of total respiratory system resistance.

The remaining 60% of total respiratory resistance is pulmonary resistance, which was assumed to be essentially the same as airway resistance and thus a reflection of airway caliber. Recent studies in dogs, however, have shown that lung tissue contributes a significant component of pulmonary resistance during constriction or bronchodilation.[21, 22]

An important factor to consider about airway resistance (Raw) is the fact that resistance to airflow is determined by the size of the airways. Airways are largest at high lung volumes and smallest at low volumes, such as residual volume. Passive changes in Raw can thus occur with changes in the lung volume in the absence of bronchodilation or constriction. Since the relationship of Raw to lung volume is not linear (Fig. 1.6), the reciprocal of Raw, conductance (Gaw), is related to lung volume in linear fashion and is used to identify the presence of bronchoconstriction or bronchodilation. Such determinants of Raw and Gaw are by convention made at FRC.

Methods of Measuring Resistance

Flow-Pressure-Volume Method. Simultaneous recordings of the three variables—flow, pressure, and tidal volume (Fig. 1.7)—provide the basis for

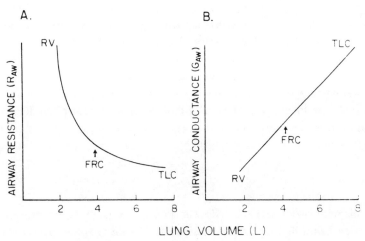

Figure 1.6. The hyperbolic relationship of airway resistance (Raw) to lung volume (**A**) is contrasted with the linear relationship (**B**) of its reciprocal airway conductance (Gaw). RV, residual volume; TLC, total lung capacity; FRC, functional residual capacity. (Reproduced with permission from Gal TJ. Pulmonary function testing. In: Miller RD, ed. Anesthesia. 3rd ed. New York: Churchill Livingstone, 1990, Chapter 24.)

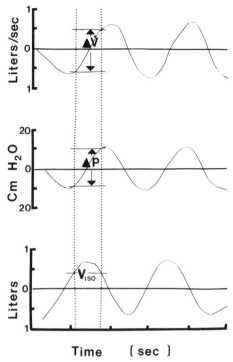

Time   [sec]

Figure 1.7.   Simultaneous record of flow ($\dot{V}$), pressure (P), and volume (V) for determination of resistance by the isovolume technique. Change in pressure (ΔP) and change in flow ($\Delta\dot{V}$) between two points where volume is identical (Viso) provides an estimate of resistance. (Reproduced with permission from Gal TJ. Monitoring the function of the respiratory system. In: Lake CL., ed. Clinical monitoring. 1st ed. Philadelphia: WB Saunders, 1989, Chapter 9.)

this analysis. The change in pressure (ΔP) and change in flow ($\Delta\dot{V}$) between two points where volume is identical (Viso) are used to calculate resistance. This method of analysis is termed the isovolume technique. Another more complex technique relating pressure flow and volume is termed the Comroe-Nisell-Nims technique.[23] With this method, static compliance is first calculated by dividing the total inspired volume by the pressure measured immediately prior to exhalation. Next, the point on the flow trace at which the expiratory flow is 0.5 liter/sec is noted and the volume of gas remaining in the lungs at this point is also measured. Dividing this volume by the compliance value gives a pressure that is associated with a flow of 0.5 liter/sec and thus provides the calculation of total respiratory resistance, whereas the use of transpulmonary pressure (PL) yields pulmonary resistance.

   Passive Exhalation Method.   The lungs fill and empty in an exponential fashion, i.e., the rate of change in the variable (lung volume) is proportional to the magnitude of the variable. Such a system can be characterized by a turnover time or time constant usually designated by the Greek letter tau (τ). The latter is the time at which volume would decrease to zero if it continued to decrease at the initial rapid rate. During one time constant, volume decreases to about 37% of its initial value or $1/e$, where $e = 2.72828$ (the base of the natural logarithm). In the respiratory system τ is equal to the product of resistance and compliance.

$$\tau(\text{sec}) = R(\text{cm H}_2\text{O}\cdot\text{liter}^{-1}\cdot\text{sec}) \times C(\text{liter}\cdot\text{cm H}_2\text{O}^{-1})$$

In this method compliance is determined in similar fashion as in the Comroe-Nissel-Nims technique, by relating ΔV (1.0 liter) to ΔP prior to exhalation. The time interval (t) to exhale to 370 ml (Fig. 1.8) is then measured to estimate the time constant (τ) of passive exhalation. This value is then divided by the compliance value to yield a calculation of total respiratory system resistance.

Forced Oscillation.   Total respiratory resistance can be measured during quiet breathing by imposing rapid small sine wave oscillations at the mouth and recording the resultant sine wave flows and pressures. Such oscillations are produced by a loudspeaker or valveless pump. To measure the pressure change due to resistance, the reactance component (i.e., that due to elastance and inertance) must be eliminated. At higher frequencies the inertial properties dominate and reactance is positive. At lower frequencies reactance is influenced by the capacity of the system (elastance) and is negative. The frequency at which reactance is zero is termed the resonant frequency of the respiratory

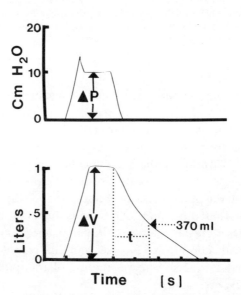

Figure 1.8.   Illustration of the passive exhalation method for estimating resistance. Compliance (C) is calculated as $\Delta V/\Delta P$ prior to exhalation. t = time constant (τ) or the time required to exhale to 37% of pre-expiratory volume (i.e., 370 ml). Resistance (R) is calculated from the equation R $\times$ C = t. (Reproduced with permission from Gal TJ. Monitoring the function of the respiratory system. In: Lake CL, ed. Clinical monitoring. 1st ed. Philadelphia: WB Saunders, 1989, Chapter 9.)

system (usually 3 to 8 Hz). At this frequency elastance and inertance are 180° out of phase (i.e., equal magnitude and opposite sign) and cancel out. The oscillating pressure wave is then due to resistance alone.[24] One of the major advantages of this technique is that it requires very little patient cooperation. However, to be a true reflection of changes in airway caliber, lung volume changes must be taken into account.

Body Plethysmography. This technique, first described by DuBois et al.,[25] has the advantage of specifically determining airway resistance (Paw) and simultaneously providing a measurement of thoracic gas volume. The patient must sit in a closed box and breathe via a mouthpiece. During panting-like breaths (2 to 3 breaths/sec), flow at the mouth measured by a pneumotachograph is displayed on the y axis of an oscilloscope, while box pressure is displayed on the x axis. The slope of this loop is usually measured between 0 and 0.5 liter/sec to compute resistance (Fig. 1.9A). When the airway is occluded

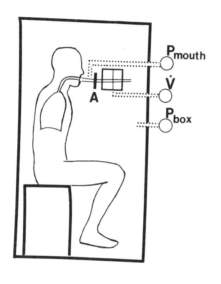

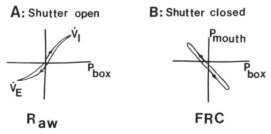

Figure 1.9. Constant-volume body plethysmograph used to determine airway resistance and thoracic gas volume by utilizing relationships of flow, box pressure, and mouth pressure during panting with shutter open (**A**) and closed (**B**). (Reproduced with permission from Gal TJ. Monitoring the function of the respiratory system. In: Lake CL, ed. Clinical monitoring. 1st ed. Philadelphia: WB Saunders, 1989, Chapter 9.)

during such panting, pressure at the mouth is displayed on the *y* axis and related to box pressure to estimate thoracic gas volume, which in most cases is the functional residual capacity (Fig. 1.9**B**) as described previously.

REFERENCES

1. Detroyer A, Estenne M. Functional anatomy of the respiratory muscles. Clin Chest Med 1988;9:175–193.
2. Hess D. History of plumonary function testing. Respir Care 1989;34:427–442.
3. Hutchinson J. On the capacity of the lungs and on the respiratory movements with the view to establishing a precise and easy method of detecting disease by the spiromenter. Lancet 1846;1:630–632.
4. Clausen JL, Zarins LP. Estimations of lung volumes from chest radiographs. In: Clausen JL, Arings LP, eds. Pulmonary function testing: guidelines and controversies. New York: Academic Press, 1982:155–163.
5. Dubois AB, Bothelo SY, Bedell GN, et al. A rapid plethysmographic method for measuring thoracic gas volume: a comparison with a nitrogen washout method for measuring functional residual capacity in normal subjects. J Clin Invest 1956;35:322–326.
6. Shore SA, Huk S, Mannix S, Martin JG. Effect of panting frequency on plethysmographic determinations of thoracic gas volume in chronic obstructive pulmonary disease. Am Rev Respir Dis 1983;128:54–59.
7. Leith DE, Mead JL. Mechanisms determining residual volume of the lungs in normal subjects. J Appl Physiol 1967;23:221–227.
8. Rahn H, Otis AB, Chadwick LE, Fenn W. The pressure volume diagram of the thorax and lung. Am J Physiol 1946;146:161–178.
9. Detroyer A, Basteiner-Geens J. Effects of neuromuscular blockade on respiratory mechanics in conscious man. J Appl Physiol 1979;47:1162–1168.
10. Gal TJ, Arora NS. Respiratory mechanics in supine subjects during partial curarization. J Appl Physiol 1986;52:57–63.
11. Agostoni E, Hyatt RE. Static behavior of the respiratory system. In: Macklem PT, Mead J, eds. Handbook of physiology, the respiratory system. Bethseda MD: American Physiological Society 1986:120.
12. Tucker DH, Sieker HO. The effect of change in body position on lung volumes and intrapulmonary gas mixing in patients with obesity, heart failure and ephysema. Am Rev Respir Dis 1960;85:787–791.
13. Scheidt M, Hyatt RE, Rehder K. Effects of rib cage or abdominal restriction of lung mechanics. J Appl Physiol 1981;51:1115–1121.
14. Agostoni E, Burtner G, Torri G, Rahn H. Respiratory mechanics during submersion and negative pressure breathing. J Appl Physiol 1966;21:251–258.
15. Koterba AM, Kosch PC, Beech J, Whitlock T. Breathing strategy of the adult horse *(Equus caballus)* at rest. J Appl Physiol 1988;64:337–346.
16. Bryan AC, Wohl MEB. Respiratory mechanics in children. In: Macklem PT, Mead J, eds. Handbook of phsyiology, the respiratory system. Bethesda MD: American Physiological Society 1986:180–181.
17. Olinsky A, Bryan MH, Bryan AC. Influence of lung inflation on respiratory control in neonates. J Appl Physiol 1974;36:426–429.
18. Colin AA, Wohl MEB, Mead J, Ratjen FA, Glass G, Stark AR. Transition from dynamically maintained to relaxed end expiratory volume in human infants. J Appl Physiol 1989;67:2107–2111.
19. Milic Emili J, Mead J, Turner JM, et al. Improved technique for estimating pleural pressure from esophageal balloons. J Apply Physiol 1964;19:207–211.
20. Leatherman NE. An improved balloon system for monitoring intraesophageal pressure in acutely ill patients. Crit Care Med 1978;6:189–192.
21. Ludwig MS, Dreshas O, Solway J, Munoz A, Ingram RH Jr. Partitioning of pulmonary resist-

ance during constriction in the dog: effect of volume history. J Appl Physiol 1987;62:807–815.

22. Warner DO, Vettermann J, Brusasco V, Rehder K. Pulmonary resistance during halothane anesthesia is not determined only by airway caliber. Anesthesiology 1989;70:453–460.

23. Comroe JH, Nisell OL, Nims RG. A simple method for concurrent measurement of compliance and resistance to breathing in anesthetized animals and man. J Appl Physiol 1954;7:225–228.

24. Fisher AG, DuBois AB, Hyde RW. Evaluation of the oscillation technique for the determination of resistance to breathing. J Clin Invest 1968;47:2045–2057.

25. DuBois AB, Bothelo SY, Comroe JH. A new method for measuring airway resistance in man using a body plethysmograph. Values in normal subjects and in patients with respiratory disease. J Clin Invest 1956;35:326–335.

Chapter 2

Physiology of Pulmonary Function Testing

Pulmonary function testing provides objective, standardized measurements for quantitating the degree of respiratory dysfunction. This is in contrast to subjective information provided by the medical history and physical examination, which seldom identify actual respiratory function abnormalities and are poor estimates of the severity of disease. This discussion concerns testing that relates to the mechanical ventilatory function of the lungs and chest wall. The cornerstone of all such testing is clinical spirometry.

CLINICAL SPIROMETRY

Vital Capacity

The most common measurement of lung function is the vital capacity (VC). This is the largest volume measured after an individual inspires deeply and maximally to total lung capacity (TLC) and then exhales completely to residual volume (RV) into a spirometer without concern for rapidity of effort (see Fig. 1.2). Normal values for VC are lower in supine subjects than in sitting subjects and vary directly with height and inversely with age. A given VC is often considered abnormal if it falls below 80% of the predicted value. Patients with an abnormally low VC are considered to have restrictive disease. The decreased VC with such restrictive disease may result from lung pathology (pneumonia, atelectasis, and pulmonary fibrosis) or may represent a loss of distensible lung tissue, as with surgical excision. Decreased VC can also occur in the absence of lung disease. In this case, muscle weakness, abdominal swelling, or pain may prevent the patient from generating either a full inspiration or a maximal expiratory effort.

Forced Expiratory Spirogram

If after a maximal inspiratory effort a subject exhales as forcefully and rapidly as possible, the maneuver is termed the forced vital capacity (FVC), and the

22

exhaled volume is recorded with respect to time. The rate of airflow during this rapid forceful exhalation indirectly reflects the flow resistance properties of the airways. In the presence of airway obstruction, FVC tends to be less than the standard slow VC because of air trapping. In healthy subjects, the two maneuvers result in nearly equal measured volumes. Since the FVC maneuver is an artificial one, patients must be instructed carefully and often require practice attempts before performing the test adequately. Generally, three acceptable tracings are required for analysis. These FVC maneuvers must be characterized by a full inspiration to TLC, followed by an abrupt onset of exhalation, and continued maximum effort throughout exhalation to RV. The exhalation should take at least 4 seconds and not be interrupted by coughing, glottic closure, or any mechanical obstruction.

The FVC is reduced by the same conditions that reduce VC. Therefore, to identify airway obstruction, flow rates are determined by calculating the volume exhaled during certain time intervals. Most commonly measured is the volume exhaled in the first second, or the forced expiratory volume in one second (FEV_1). The FEV_1 is expressed as absolute volume in liters or as a percentage of the forced vital capacity ($FEV_1/FVC\%$). For the purposes of reporting and calculating values, the largest observed FVC and FEV_1 from any of the three acceptable spirograms are used even if they are not obtained from the same curve.[1] Normal healthy subjects can exhale 75 to 80% of their FVC in the first second; the remaining volume is exhaled in 2 or 3 additional seconds (Fig.

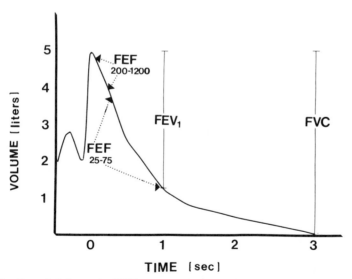

Figure 2.1.   Forced vital capacity (FVC) maneuver in a normal subject. Exhaled volume is plotted against time as the subject expires forcefully, rapidly, and completely to residual volume (RV) following a maximal deep inspiration. FEV_1, forced expired volume in 1 second; $FEF_{200-1200}$, forced expiratory flow between 200 and 1200 ml of expired volume; $FEF_{25-75\%}$, forced expiratory flow over the midportion of vital capacity, that is, from 25 to 75% of expired volume.

2.1). Diseases such as asthma and bronchitis, which produce airway obstruction, reduce expiratory flow rate and thus reduce FEV_1 and $FEV_1/FVC\%$. Restrictive diseases are not usually associated with airway obstruction but do cause decreases in FVC. Although the absolute volume of FEV_1 may be reduced on a similar basis, the FEV_1 expressed as a percentage of FVC is usually normal (i.e., $FEV_1/FVC > 70\%$).

The maximal flow rate obtainable at any time during an FVC manuever is termed the peak flow, which is measured in liters per second or liters per minute. Peak flow can be measured by drawing a tangent to the steepest part of the FVC spirogram, but this is subject to large errors. More commonly, maximal flow is measured as the average flow during the liter of gas expired after the initial 200 ml during an FVC maneuver (Fig. 2.1). This is usually designated as forced expiratory flow ($FEF_{200-1200}$), although the term maximal expiratory flow rate (MEFR) has been used in the past. This flow is slightly lower than the true peak flow, which can be measured conveniently with a hand-held flowmeter or more accurately with a pneumotachograph. Peak flow is markedly affected by obstruction of large airways and is particularly responsive to bronchodilator therapy. Since repeat measurements are convenient to obtain, peak flow rates can be used to monitor therapeutic responses in acute asthma. Normal values in healthy males under 40 years of age are typically greater than 500 liters/min. Values less than 200 liters/min in the surgical candidate suggest impaired cough efficiency and the high likelihood of postoperative complications.[2] The test is less unpleasant and exhausting for patients than the FVC maneuver and thus provides a valuable tool to identify gross pulmonary disability at the bedside.

Because peak flow is highly dependent on patient effort, the measurement may vary with effort and not solely reflect airway function. In contrast, high degrees of expiratory effort are not required to achieve maximal flow at intermediate and low lung volumes. Therefore, flow is often measured over the middle half of the FVC (i.e., between 25 and 75% of expired volume). This parameter, formerly called the maximal mid-expiratory flow, is now referred to as the forced mid-expiratory flow ($FEF_{25-75\%}$). Since the flow does not include the initial highly effort-dependent portion of forced expiration, $FEF_{25-75\%}$ is often referred to as effort independent. This designation is not entirely appropriate, since $FEF_{25-75\%}$ can be decreased by marked reductions in expiratory effort and by a submaximal inspiration preceding the FVC maneuver. The term "effort independent" is used rather to signify that above a certain modest effort, additionally increased effort has no effect in increasing flow any further. The same flow rates may also decrease with truly maximal effort compared to slightly suboptimal effort.[3] This phenomenon has been termed "negative effort dependence" and appears to be in part an artifact of measuring volume changes at the mouth rather than actual changes in thoracic gas volume. It probably also reflects the marked airway compression associated with truly maximal effort.

Values for $FEF_{25-75\%}$ in healthy young men average 4.5 to 5.0 liters/sec. However, because of the wide variations among normal subjects the predicted limits of normal may be as low as 2 liters/sec. The measurement has often been proposed as a sensitive test for mild obstruction in the small airways, but it has been shown that patients undergoing spirometric testing for suspected airway obstruction seldom had abnormal values for $FEF_{25-75\%}$ when FEV_1/FEV was 75% or greater.[4] Thus, the $FEF_{25-75\%}$ does not appear to be more sensitive than FEV_1 in detecting minor abnormalities of the spirogram.

MAXIMUM VOLUNTARY VENTILATION

Dynamic lung function is also evaluted by measuring the maximum breathing capacity or, more specifically, the maximum voluntary ventilation (MVV). This is the largest volume that can be breathed per minute by voluntary effort. The patient is instructed to breathe as hard and fast as possible for 12 seconds. The measured volume is then extrapolated to 1 minute and expressed as liters per minute. Since high rates of airflow are required, the MVV is significantly affected by changes in airway resistance. MVV is usually reduced in patients with obstructive airway disease and correlates well with FEV_1 measured in liters ($FEV_1 \times 35$ approximates MVV). Discrepancies between the measured MVV and that predicted by FEV_1 often reflect patient effort. The MVV as a comprehensive test of ventilatory function is altered by factors other than airway obstruction. These include the elastic properties of the lung and chest wall, respiratory muscle strength, learning, coordination, and motivation. In healthy male adults MVV averages 150 to 175 liters/min. This extremely high level of ventilatory effort cannot be maintained for much longer than 1 minute. However, approximately 80% of the MVV can be maintained by healthy subjects for as long as 15 minutes, and up to 60% of MVV can be sustained for even longer periods. Abnormally low values (less than 80% of predicted) do not identify specific defects but do indicate gross impairment in respiratory function. The test has a unique value in the surgical candidate because of its dependence on intangible variables such as cooperation, motivation, and stamina.

RESPIRATORY MUSCLE STRENGTH

All of the previously mentioned measurements of pulmonary function that require patient effort are influenced by the strength of the respiratory muscles. The latter can be specifically evaluated by measurement of maximal static respiratory pressures. The pressures are generated against an occluded airway during a maximal forced inspiratory or expiratory effort and are usually measured with simple aneroid gauges.[5] Maximal static inspiratory pressure Pımax) is measured when inspiratory muscles are at their optimal length near RV (Fig. 2.2). Similarly, maximal static expiratory pressure (Pᴇmax is measured when expiratory muscles are optimally stretched after a full inspiration to near TLC.

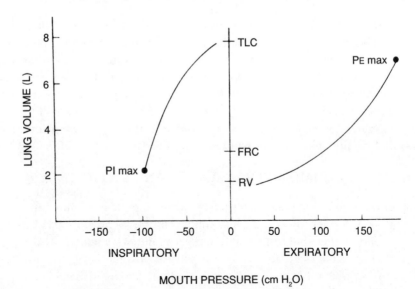

Figure 2.2. Typical values for maximum static inspiratory (PImax) and expiratory (PEmax) pressures measured at the mouth are plotted as a function of lung volume from residual volume (RV) to total lung capacity. (Reproduced with permission from Gal TJ. Pulmonary function testing. In: Miller RD, ed. Anesthesia. 3rd ed. New York: Churchill Livingstone, 1990, Chapter 24.)

In young adult males PImax is about $(-)125$ cm H_2O and PEmax is about $(+)200$ cm H_2O.

Thus, pressures measured at the mouth include that generated by the respiratory muscles and a portion resulting from the elastic recoil of the respiratory system. The latter is essentially zero at functional residual capacity (FRC). Pressures measured at FRC are slightly less than at the extremes of lung volume (Fig. 2.2) but, unlike the other values, reflect solely the pressure developed by the respiratory muscles.

A PImax of $(-)25$ cm H_2O or lower indicates severe inability to take a deep breath, while a PEmax of lower than $(+)40$ cm H_2O suggests severely impaired coughing ability. Although these pressures are not measured routinely in all pulmonary function laboratories, they are particularly useful in evaluating patients with neuromuscular disorders. In these patients, the vital capacity has long been used to indicate the severity of respiratory muscle weakness and predict respiratory failure. Measurements of respiratory muscle strength have been shown to identify more readily the patients in whom respiratory muscle weakness is the primary cause of hypercapneic respiratory failure.[6]

PHYSIOLOGICAL DETERMINANTS OF MAXIMUM FLOW RATES

The maximal flow rates that can be achieved during pulmonary function testing depend on three factors, each of which is highly dependent on the volume of the lung at the time. One of these factors is the degree of effort, or the driving pressure generated by muscle contraction. The expiratory effort reflected by PEmax is maximal at high lung volumes near TLC and decreases as lung volume decreases (Fig. 2.2). Maximal inspiratory effort (PImax), on the other hand, is achieved at low lung volumes near RV and diminishes at high lung volumes.

Another important determinant of flow is the elastic recoil pressure of the lung (PL). At all lung volumes from RV to TLC, the lung has a tendency to recoil inward (see Fig. 1.3). The PL, therefore, is greatest at TLC (25 to 30 cm H_2O) and lowest at RV (2 to 3 cm H_2O). This PL tends to augment flows during expiration and acts to oppose flow during inspiration. The PL is opposed by the outward recoil of the chest wall (Pcw) except at very high lung volumes. The recoil pressure of the respiratory system (Prs) is the algebraic sum of PL + Pcw. Note again that PL and Pcw are equal and opposite (i.e., Prs = 0) at FRC, which is the resting volume of the respiratory system.

The final factor, which opposes these two driving pressures, is the resistance to flow provided by the airways. This airway resistance (Raw) is determined by the size of the airways. Since airways are largest at high lung volumes and smallest at RV, Raw is greatest at RV and least at TLC (see Fig. 1.6A).

Flow-Volume Relationships

Since all the determinants of maximal flow are dependent on lung volume, a useful format to assess the flow-resistive properties of the airways is to plot flow as a function of volume during the forced vital capacity maneuver. At the beginning of the forced expiration, the rate of flow quickly rises to a maximal or peak value at a lung volume near TLC. As expiration continues, lung volume decreases, airways narrow, resistance increases, and the flow rates progressively decrease. The impact of obstructive airway disease on such flow rates is emphasized in Figure 2.3. In patients with airway obstruction, flows are reduced over the full range of lung volume from TLC to RV.

The influence of expiratory effort on the flow-volume curves is very important. An individual can actually inscribe different flow-volume curves with differing efforts, although each may have the same FVC (Fig. 2.4). At large lung volumes close to TLC, airflow rises with increasing effort (curve *A*). Curves *B* and *C* with decreasing effort exhibit decreased flows in this high range of lung volume, but all three curves merge at a point and continue together to RV. At these intermediate and low lung volumes, only moderate effort is needed to produce maximal flow. Since increased expiratory effort has little effect on increasing these flows, there is little difference between the three curves and this portion of the curve is referred to as effort independent. At this point, flow is largely a function of the other two variables (PL and Raw). Once again it is important to point out that exaggerated effort may decrease these same flows, as is the case with FEV_1 and $FEF_{25-75\%}$.[7]

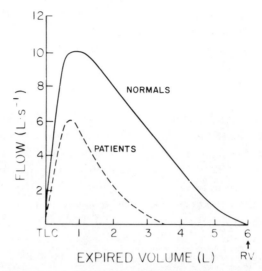

Figure 2.3.   Maximum expiratory flow-volume curves in normals contrasted with those typically seen in patients with obstructive airway disease. Expiratory flow is plotted as a function of lung volume during maximal expiration from total lung capacity (TLC) to residual volume (RV). (Reproduced with permission from Gal TJ. Pulmonary function testing. In: Miller RD, ed. Anesthesia. 3rd ed. New York: Churchill Livingstone, 1990, Chapter 24.)

The rate of airflow during forced expiration is influenced not only by the effort expended but also by the lung volume at which the expiratory maneuver is begun. True maximum flows occur only when expiration is begun at or near TLC. When forced expirations are begun with maximal effort from volumes below TLC (Fig. 2.5), peak flow is not as high but flows quickly and conforms

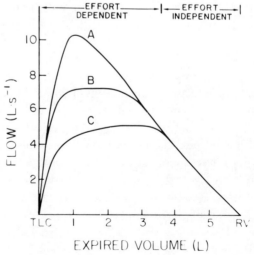

Figure 2.4.   Forced expiratory flow-volume curves in a normal subject. The exhalation from total lung capacity (TLC) to residual volume (RV) was performed at three levels of effort ranging from maximal (*A*) to minimal (*C*). (Reproduced with permission from Gal TJ. Pulmonary function testing. In: Miller RD, ed. Anesthesia. 3rd ed. New York: Churchill Livingstsone, 1990, Chapter 24.)

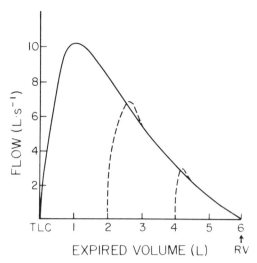

Figure 2.5. Expiratory flow-volume curves produced by maximal effort with exhalation begun at total lung capacity (TLC) and 2 and 4 liters below TLC. (Reproduced with permission from Gal TJ. Pulmonary function testing. In: Miller RD, ed. Anesthesia. 3rd ed. New York: Churchill Livingstone, 1990, Chapter 24.)

to the same performance envelope as if the maneuvers were begun at TLC. Even healthy subjects can exhibit a decreased FEV_1/FVC ratio when the forced expirations are started from such submaximal volumes. Therein lies some of the advantage of a flow-volume plot as opposed to the volume-time tracing with conventional spirometry.

Flow Limitation during Maximal Expiration

The failure of increasing effort to further augment flow over the lower two-thirds of the vital capacity results from dynamic compression of the airways. This mechanism, which normally limits flows, is illustrated by a model of the lung in which the alveoli can be considered as elastic sacs and the intrathoracic airways as a collapsible tube with both enclosed in the pleural cavity. This model of flow limitation is often termed the equal pressure point (EPP) theory. The pressure head that serves to move air from the alveoli to the mouth is provided by the alveolar pressure (Pa). At any given lung volume when there is no flow, such as end inspiration (Fig. 2.6A), pleural pressure (Pp1) is subatmospheric and counterbalances lung recoil pressure (PL). Thus, the sum of the two pressures, Pa, is zero, as are pressures at the mouth and through the remaining airways. During forced expiration (Fig. 2.6**B**), Pp1 rises above atmospheric (becomes positive). The increased Pa is again the sum of PL + Pp1. Pressure is dissipated along the airway in overcoming resistance to flow and finally reaches zero at the mouth. At some point along the airway, the intraluminal pressure falls to a level that equals the surrounding pleural pressure. This site is referred to as the equal pressure point (EPP). Toward the mouth (downstream) the lateral pressure within the airway lumen is less than the com-

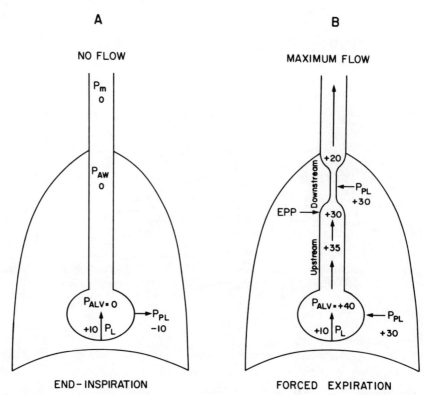

Figure 2.6.   Model of expiratory flow limitation using the equal pressure point (EPP) theory. Mouth pressure (Pm), intraluminal airway pressure (Paw), lung elastic recoil pressure (PL), pleural pressure (Ppl), and alveolar pressure (Palv) are depicted at the end of a quiet inspiration (**A**) with cessation of flow and with maximal flows during forced expiration (**B**). (Reproduced with permission from Gal TJ. Pulmonary function testing. In: Miller RD, ed. Anesthesia. 3rd ed. New York: Churchill Livingstone, 1990, Chapter 24.)

pression Ppl, and the airways tend to collapse. Once maximal flow is reached, further increases in Ppl from increasing effort do not affect airflow in the upstream segment (from EPP toward the alveoli), since the driving pressure along this portion of the airway is essentially equal to PL. Therein lies the origin of the term "effort independent." The increase in Ppl simply produces more compression of the downstream airways (from EPP to mouth). Thus, increasing effort augments airway compression but fails to increase flow.

The principal value of this dynamic airway compression is in the production of an effective cough. Even though maximum flows may not be reached, the compressed downstream airway develops an increased linear velocity of airflow, which maximizes the removal of secretions along airway walls. At intermediate lung volumes EPPs lie in segmental bronchi, but they may move farther upstream toward the alveoli at lower lung volumes. The dynamic compression involves primarily lobar and mainstem bronchi and the intrathoracic trachea. Coughing is therefore most effective in removing material from these relatively large airways.

Mechanisms of Decreased Airflow in Disease

Abnormal expiratory flow rates may be seen in many disease states and may result from alterations in any of the three major deterinants of flow (P_{E}max, P_L, and Raw). For example, patients with neuromuscular disease who may exhibit decreased expiratory flows include those with myasthenia gravis, muscular dystrophy, Guillain-Barré syndrome, or spinal cord transection. Decreased ability to generate expiratory effort is the principal cause of low expiratory flows in these patients, who seldom exhibit increases in Raw or decreased P_L. Other categories of restrictive disease, such as musculoskeletal deformities (kyphoscoliosis, ankylosing spondylitis, and interstitial lung disease), are often associated with near-normal muscle strength. In these situations, expiratory flows may actually be slightly increased because of an increased P_L associated with reductions in lung volume. Reduced lung volumes associated with long-term neuromuscular disease may likewise be associated with increases in P_L, which may result in more normal expiratory flow rates.

The classic example of decreased expiratory flow associated with decreased lung recoil (P_L) is in emphysema. Here, expiratory muscle strength is usually adequate and lung distention tends to increase airway size, such that Raw is also usually normal. In patients with bronchitis and asthma, on the other hand, airway narrowing is prominent. In these two variants of obstructive lung disease the major factor reducing flow is an increased Raw. Early changes in these obstructive lung diseases are often confined to the peripheral airways. Narrowing in these airways does produce reduced expiratory flows at mid and low lung volumes but does not appreciably affect measurements in Raw or the other determinants of airflow.

MEASUREMENT OF AIRWAY OBSTRUCTION

Airway Resistance

Of the standard techniques used to evaluate airway obstruction, airway resistance (Raw) measurements appear to be the most sensitive and direct. The technique is rapid, noninvasive, and merely requires that a subject pant once or twice per second through a mouthpiece and with a nose clip in place. During normal breathing a major fraction of the resistance to airflow resides in the nose, pharynx, and larynx and can mask changes taking place in the lungs. The use of a mouthpiece bypasses the nose to minimize the effects of the upper airway on the measurement. The panting maneuver is likewise used to keep the larynx dilated and reduce its influence on the total resistance to airflow. The measurement of Raw requires the subject to sit in a constant-volume body plethysmograph ("body box") that also permits the recording of thoracic gas volume, and thereby provides an accurate appraisal of the effect of lung volume on Raw. Lung volume is estimated by using Boyle's law to relate changes in box pressure and mouth pressure, while Raw is calculated from changes in box pressure and flow. The subjects initially pant against a closed mouthpiece, usually at end expiration. Thus, thoracic gas volume (FRC) is calculated from the relationship of box pressure to mouth pressure (see Fig. 1.9). The shutter in the mouthpiece is then opened, and continued panting inscribes the relationship between box pressure and flow at the mouth to drive Raw. The upper limit of normal Raw is usually considered to be 2 cm $H_2O \cdot liter^{-1} \cdot sec$. To eliminate passive changes in Raw as a result of difference in lung volume, the reciprocal of Raw, airway conductance (Gaw), is calculated. This Gaw is usually divided by the lung volume at which the measurement is made (usually FRC) to obtain specific airway conductance (sGaw). The coefficient of variation (standard deviation/mean $\times$ 100) in normal baseline values for the same subject is usually small (less than 10%). Therefore, sGaw is a highly reproducible measurement that can identify changes in the caliber of the intrapulmonary airways. However, a significant portion of normal airway resistance resides in the upper airways. Since the latter can be significantly affected by head flexion,[8] it is important that patients position themselves as erect as possible when attached to the mouthpiece in the body box.

Forced Expiratory Maneuvers

Despite the specificity and sensitivity of Raw measurements, airway obstruction is more commonly evaluated by measurement of maximal forced expiration, since the latter requires less complex equipment. The indices obtained from forced expiration, unlike Raw, are determined by a complex interrelationship between the flow-resistive properties of intrathoracic airways and the elastic recoil of the lung. The simplest of such measurements is the peak expiratory flow, which is conveniently measured with a variable-orifice flow meter. Since the peak flow occurs early in a forced expiration, flow limitation has not occurred in the airways and, thus, flow is highly dependent on effort and subject cooperation. However, since the variation for the measurement in the same subject is surprisingly low, peak expiratory flow is a fairly reproducible test of airway function.

Another extensively used indirect measure of airway dimensions is the FEV_1. Again, during the first 25% of a forced vital capacity maneuver, flow reflects dimensions of the airways between the alveoli and the mouth and is effort dependent. Although the physiological parameters governing the remaining flow are complex, FEV_1, like peak flow, is simple and reproducible and is thus a useful index of airway function. The measurement is subject to day-to-day variability, which is greater in patients with obstructive airway disease than in normal persons.[9] Thus, changes in FEV_1 must exceed 15% to signify bronchodilation or constriction. The same varability applies to measurements of $FEF_{25-75\%}$. In addition, one must account for the possibilities of negative effort dependence[7] and, more importantly, the changes in FVC that might occur. For example, in the case of bronchodilation, FVC may increase but actually produce a misleading decrease in $FEF_{25-75\%}$.[10] Thus the measurement should be adjusted to the same absolute lung volume, i.e., the same segment of FVC below total lung capacity.

Additional assessment of the flow-resistive properties of the airways can be obtained from maximal expiratory flow-volume (MEFV) curves, which illustrate the relationship between airflow and lung volume during a forced vital capacity maneuver. A typical response when bronchoconstriction is induced consists of diminished flows throughout the whole MEFV curve envelope (Fig. 2.3). Ventilatory flows and FVC usually decrease, while RV increases. Therefore, expiratory flows must be measured at the same reference lung volume. This is usually at a fixed percentage of the baseline or normal FVC and requires that all curves be superimposed at TLC.

In normal subjects, full inflation to TLC may remove the bronchoconstriction induced by mechanical stimuli or drugs, while in asthmatics an increase in bronchomotor tone may accompany the same deep inspiration. To overcome these variable effects of a full inspiration on bronchial tone, Bouhuys and coworkers propsed that flows be measured with partial expiratory flow-volume (PEFV) curves.[11] In this case, the maximal forced expiration is started at or slightly above the middle of FVC. In all cases, the PEFV curve is followed by a full inhalation to TLC and a maximal forced exhalation to RV to obtain a reference MEFV curve. Flows are usually measured between 20 and 40% of VC above RV. Since PEFV curves are unaffected by change in upper airway resistance, they are sensitive to the changes in the intrapulmonary airways and have been suggested as a useful alternative to Raw for detecting bronchoconstrictor and bronchodilator responses, and are particularly useful in normal subjects.

Flow-Volume Loops

Reductions in peak flow, MVV, and FEV_1 without additional clinical evidence of chronic obstructive lung disease may indicate the presence of an obstructing lesion of the upper airway, larynx, or trachea. This obstruction may be suspected by a careful history and physical examination but often simulates diffuse airway obstruction and suggests a marked degree of lung dysfunction. This is most likely to occur in patients for head and neck surgery who may present for operative procedures related to these lesions. Flow-volume (F-V) loops provide a graphic analysis of flow at various lung volumes and have been used to determine whether or not patients have upper airway obstructive lesions. Both flow and volume are plotted simultaneously on an x-y recorder as subjects inhale fully to total lung capacity (TLC) and then perform an FVC maneuver. This is followed immediately by a maximal inspiration as quickly as possible back to TLC (Fig. 2.7). Note that expiratory flow decreases over the latter half of the exhaled volume (Fig. 2.7**A**) despite the sustained expiratory effort indicated by the high positive pleural pressure (Fig. 2.7**B**). During maximal inspiration, airways do not undergo compression. Rather, with increasing inspiratory effort, airways become distended by the subatmospheric (negative) pleural

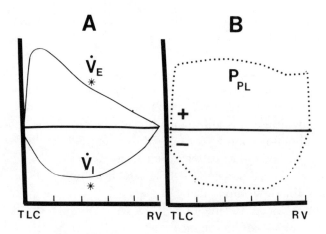

LUNG VOLUME [L]

Figure 2.7. **A,** Schematic representation of maximum inspiratory ($\dot{V}_I$) and expiratory ($\dot{V}_E$) flows plotted as a function of lung volume loop. **B,** Pleural pressure (Ppl) plotted as a function of lung volume from total lung capacity (TLC) to residual volume (RV). The asterisk denotes flow at the midpoint (50%) of vital capacity, i.e., $\dot{V}_{I50}$ and $\dot{V}_{E50}$.

pressure, and flow is increased. Thus, the entire inspiratory portion of the loop (as well as the expiratory curve near TLC) is highly dependent on effort. The ratio of expiratory flow to inspiratory flow at 50% of vital capacity (mid-VC ratio) is normally about 1.0. This ratio is particularly useful in identifying the presence of upper airway obstruction, in which case inspiratory flow tends to be reduced more than expiratory flow, and the mid-VC ratio is increased, i.e., greater than 1.

Flow-volume loops not only aid in suggesting upper airway obstruction but may help to localize the site and nature of the obstruction. Several character-istic patterns have been described.[12] Perhaps the most common lesion is a fixed obstruction such as a benign stricture resulting from tracheostomy or tracheal intubation. A tumor or mass such as a goiter may also produce a similar pic-ture, as would breathing through a fixed external resistance. No significant change in airway diameter occurs during inspiration or expiration. As a result, expiratory flows show a plateau of constant flow over the effort-dependent portion of vital capacity. Inspiratory flows show a similar pleateau (Fig. 2.8**A**). Since both are reduced to nearly the same extent, the mid-VC ratio remains approximately 1.0.

A lesion whose influence varies with the phase of respiration is termed a variable obstruction. Variable extrathoracic obstructions (Fig. 2.8**B**) are most commonly associated with vocal cord paralysis, which is usually accompanied by inspiratory stridor. A similar pattern may be seen with marked pharyngeal muscle weakness in curarized volunteers[13] and in persons with chronic neu-romuscular disorders.[14] The flow pattern has also been noted occasionally in

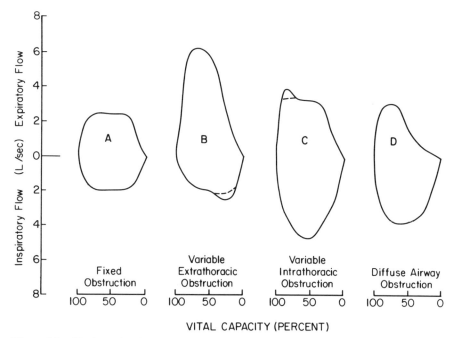

Figure 2.8. Maximum inspiratory and expiratory flow-volume curves (flow-volume loops) in four varieties of airway obstruction. (Reproduced with permission from Gal TJ. Pulmonary function testing. In: Miller RD, ed. Anesthesia. 3rd ed. New York: Churchill Livingstone, 1990, Chapter 24.)

patients with severe obstructive sleep apnea. During forced inspiration, the negative transmural pressure inside the airway tends to collapse the airway with increasing effort and thus reduces inspiratory flow. During expiration the positive pressure within the upper airway tends to decrease the obstruction so that expiratory flow is reduced far less and may even be normal. The mid-VC ratio of expiratory to inspiratory flow is often greater than 2.0.

The other form of variable obstruction occurs intrathoracically and is usually due to tumors of the trachea or major bronchi. During forced expiration, the high pleural pressures decrease airway diameter and may increase the obstruction. A plateau flow usually occurs during expiration when the compressed airway lumen assumes its minimal size at the area of the lesion (Fig. 2.8**C**). During inspiration the lowered pleural pressure surrounding the airway tends to decrease the obstruction, such that the inspiratory portion of the flow-volume loop may be quite normal. The mid-VC ratio of expiratory to inspiratory flow is low as in the case of diffuse airway obstruction (Fig. 2.8**D**). However, the shapes of the curves differ. Curve **D,** an example of diffuse airway obstruction, exhibits abnormal decreased flow in the segment near residual volume. Curve **C,** on the other hand, demonstrates normal flow in this area.

The physiological diagnosis of upper airway obstruction is sometimes difficult in patients with diffuse airway obstruction such as chronic bronchitis or asthma. These conditions themselves produce significant abnormalities of the flow-volume loop (Fig. 2.8**D**). Therefore, flow-volume loops will most clearly identify upper airway obstruction in the absence of significant generalized airway disease.

PULMONARY FUNCTION TESTING IN SURGICAL PATIENTS

Pulmonary function testing has assumed an increasing role in the preoperative preparation of many surgical patients. Such preoperative screening is aimed at identifying individuals with abnormal lung function in hopes of altering their outcome by reducing the risk of postoperative ventilatory impairment and respiratory complications. Clinically important abnormalities in pulmonary function occur in many surgical patients and include such phenomena as reduced lung volumes, rapid shallow breathing, and impaired gas exchange. These alterations in pulmonary function may be induced by the anesthetic, the surgical procedure, the associated body position, or medications administered immediately postoperatively. It has been suggested that these changes, which occur in normal patients, may be more severe in patients who undergo surgery with compromised pulmonary function and thus lead to postoperative pulmonary complications. Such complications usually include bronchospasm, bronchitis and purulent sputum, disabling cough, pneumonia, and respiratory failure as indicated by abnormal blood gases.

Although there is no general agreement concerning which particular patients should be studied preoperatively, the following types of patients are usually considered candidates for screening of preoperative pulmonary function:

1. Patients with any evidence of chronic pulmonary disease;
2. Heavy smokers, especially those with a history of persistent cough;
3. Patients with chest wall and spinal deformities;
4. Morbidly obese patients;
5. Elderly patients (more than 70 years of age);
6. Patients for thoracic surgery; and
7. Patients for upper abdominal surgery.

Initial identification of most of these patients is accomplished by history, physical examination, and chest x-rays. The question then arises as to which pulmonary function studies are appropriate for preoperative evaluation. The objective of testing in the preoperative setting is not to detect mild early lung disease, but rather to predict the likelihood of pulmonary complications. No single test appears to be the best predictor of risk. The optimal scheme for evaluating patients preoperatively is by means of arterial blood gas analysis and clinical spirometry. The FEV_1, FVC, FVC_1/FVC%, peak flow, and forced mid-expiratory flow can be obtained from a single spirometric study.

The decision about whether the observed values in a given patient are normal or abnormal requires comparing the measured values with predicted standard reference values. The most widely used normal standards are values reported by Morris et al.[15] These were determined from measurements in 1000 healthy nonsmokers residing in a relatively pollution-free environment. Normal limits are set by regression equations derived from studies such as those in large groups of normal subjects. An acceptable method to establish normal limits for general use is to define the lower limit of normal as a point $1.64 \times$ SEE (the standard deviation of the regression line) below the mean value for the same age and height on the regression line. With this approach 95% of the normal population should fall within the normal range. The widely used convention of setting lower limits of normal at 80% of the predicted value should be avoided.[16]

Abnormalities on spirometric tests have been shown to correlate with the incidence of postoperative pulmonary complications.[2] However, it must be emphasized that the incidence and severity of postoperative pulmonary complications are not directly related to the severity of preoperative lung dysfunction. The site of the surgical incision is probably far more important, since upper abdominal and thoracic surgery are associated with far more frequent problems. Obesity, patient age, and extent of smoking history are of considerable importance also.

The emphasis on evaluating preoperative pulmonary function is largely based on predicting the risk of postoperative complications. The identification of abnormal lung function, in particular obstructive airway disease, is also important to reduce intraoperative and anesthetic morbidity. A reduced FEV_1/FVC, for example, not only documents the presence of airway obstruction but also suggests the likelihood of increased airway reactivity. The site and nature of many surgical procedures often provide very little latitude for choosing between regional and general anesthesia. In patients with airway obstruction and irritable airways, instrumentation such as laryngoscopy and endotracheal intubation is fraught with the hazard of provoking reflex bronchoconstriction, particularly under light anesthesia. In many patients with obstructive airway disease the deep levels of inhalation anesthesia required to blunt airway reflexes[17] are difficult to achieve because of poor ventilation-perfusion matching. Furthermore, if achieved they are poorly tolerated by the cardiovascular system. Thus it is important to use prophylactic measures to minimize airway response. These may include anticholinergics and β-agonists inhaled as aerosols preopoeratively and intravenous opioids and lidocaine prior to airway instrumentation.

Patients with an abnormally low FEV_1 preoperatively are likely to develop severe hypercapnia when allowed to breathe spontaneously under general anesthesia. The magnitude of the CO_2 rise is directly related to the reduction in FEV_1.[18] It therefore appears prudent to control ventilation in such patients. With controlled ventilation low inspiratory flow rates were thought to be necessary with such obstruction to minimize peak airway pressures and hence pulmonary barotrauma and circulatory disturbances. Recent studies,[19, 20] however, have shown that a high inspiratory flow rate in such patients produced improved gas exchange and was not complicated by barotrauma or circulatory depression. An important consequence of the increased inspiratory flow rate was a reduced total inspiratory time (including pause). Consequently, increased time was allowed for exhalation. This increased expiratory time allows more complete emptying of alveoli, which must empty through high-resistance airways. Conversely, with a shorter expiratory time necessitated by a lower inspiratory flow, these alveoli neither empty completely nor receive as much air at the same distending pressures. In addition to all of these considerations, the anesthetic technique should ideally be tailored to allow prompt awakening at the end of the operation with as few sequelae as possible and minimal residual anesthesia.

EVALUATION OF THE PATIENT FOR LUNG RESECTION

Resection of lung tissue results in a greater impairment in postoperative lung function than most other types of surgery. These patients require a more extensive pulmonary evaluation, particularly if removal of an entire lung is anticipated. A major aim of the evaluation is to decide whether the resectional surgery can be tolerated without compromising pulmonary function to a degree that the patient dies of pulmonary insufficiency or is severely disabled. The long-term ability to withstand such lung resection relates to the amount and functional status of the lung parenchyma removed and more importantly to the function of the remaining lung tissue. Removal of lung from an already compromised patient may be followed by inadequate gas exchange, pulmonary hypertension, and an incapacitating degree of dyspnea.

Although much of the emphasis in this area deals with long-term disability in the pneumonectomy patient, it is important to note that in patients undergoing lobectomy the immediate impact on pulmonary function may be as great because of surgical trauma to the remaining tissue of the same lung. The pulmonary function studies must be viewed in light of the patient's age, status of the cardiovascular system, and cooperation and motivation. Data from pneumonectomy patients indicate that whole-lung removal will be tolerated if the preoperative pulmonary function meets the following criteria:[21] (*a*) FEV_1 greater than 2 liters and FEV_1/FVC ratio of at least 50%, (*b*) MVV greater than 50% of predicted, (*c*) ratio of residual volume to total lung capacity less than 50%.

If any of these criteria are not met, more sophisticated testing of split lung function is indicated. Usually, these tests consist of xenon radiospirometry to assess ventilation and macroaggregates of iodine or technetium to scan perfusion. The relative contribution of each lung to either total ventilation or perfusion can then be used to predict postoperative pulmonary function. A predicted postoperative FEV_1 of at least 800 ml is required before allowing pneumonectomy. The risk of significant resting CO_2 retention appears to be high with FEV_1 values less than this. If surgery is still contemplated in the face of this low predicted FEV_1, further invasive study is recommended. The pulmonary artery of the lung to be removed is subjected to occlusion by a balloon. If pulmonary hypertension (mean pulmonary arterial pressure greater than 35 mm Hg) and arterial hypoxemia (Pao_2 less than 45 mm Hg) do not occur, it is concluded that the remaining lung may be able to accommodate the entire cardiac output. Such a patient may be allowed to undergo surgery in spite of failure to fulfill the mechanical ventilatory criteria. The indications for performing this invasive procedure are not agreed on universally, but Olsen et al.[21] feel that balloon occlusion, if feasible, should be done when the less invasive studies are inconclusive.

The accuracy of predicting postpneumonectomy FEV_1 with split lung function testing has been at times disappointing and inaccurate and may not be the best way of predicting postoperative cardiopulmonary function.[22] The primary advantage of such testing is the low level of invasiveness compared to pulmonary artery occlusion and bronchospirometry, which radiospirometry essentially supplanted. The latter may in turn be supplanted by preoperative studies of exercise capacity. Recent observations suggest that a patient's maximal oxygen uptake during exercise (Vo_2max) was an accurate means of preoperatively identifying patients likely to develop postthoracotomy morbidity.[23] Thus, many patients who otherwise might have been considered inoperable on the basis of FEV_1 values might be considered to be operative candidates because of their performance and high Vo_2max during exercise. Conversely, patients with marked reductions in exercise Vo_2 preoperatively appear to be at high risk of postoperative morbidity regardless of the degree of impairment on routine and split-function pulmonary testing.

PREOPERATIVE MEASURES TO IMPROVE LUNG FUNCTION

The basic goal of preoperative pulmonary function testing is to alter outcome by reducing the morbidity and mortality associated with postoperative pulmonary complications. The assumption is that the patients identified as abnormal may benefit from therapeutic measures to improve lung function and thus reduce the likelihood of postoperative complications. Several groups have applied such therapy to poor-risk patients and produced a decrease in the postoperative complications to levels approaching those found in patients with normal lung function.[24–26]

Usually the therapy is carried out for 48 to 72 hours prior to surgery. However, it is equally important that the measures be continued postoperatively as well. Although a detailed discussion of such prophylaxis and therapy is beyond the scope of this presentation, the treatment regimen is aimed largely at removing secretions, eliminating infection, and reversing bronchospasm. It appears unreasonable to expect more than a slight reversal in airflow obstruction and arterial blood gases in stable patients with such a 48- to 72-hour regimen. Gracey et al.[27] attempted to improve pulmonary function preoperatively in patients with chronic obstructive pulmonary disease with such a standardized regimen. Although this therapy produced statistically significant changes in several tests of pulmonary function, the functional significance of the changes was doubtful. Nevertheless, the incidence of complications was dramatically reduced as in other studies. There are no definitive data that can identify whether this reduced complication rate results specifically from the preparation regimen, use of specific agents or techniques, or just the added attention paid to patients with identified airway obstruction.

It appears reasonably well established that patients whose clinical history and physical examination suggest the presence of pulmonary disease are at increased risk if spirometric testing is abnormal. It is far from clear exactly what should be done for such patients with abnormal test results short of an abbreviated regimen of preoperative preparation and concern intraopoeratively for controlling airway reactivity. Equally uncertain is which test best predicts risk and what further testing is appropriate for patients with abnormal spirometry, particularly those about to undergo pulmonary resection.

REFERENCES

1. American Thoracic Society. Standardization of spirometry. 1987 Update. Am Rev Respir Dis 1987;136:1285–2198.
2. Stein M, Koota GM, Simon M, Frank HA. Pulmonary evaluation of surgical patients. JAMA 1962;181:765–770.
3. Suratt PM, Hooe DM, Owens DA, Antharvedi A. Effect of maximal versus submaximal expiratory effort on spirometric values. Respiration 1981;42:233–236.
4. Gelb AF, Williams AJ, Zamel N. Spirometry FEV_1 vs 25–75 percent. Chest 1983;84:473–474.
5. Black LF, Hyatt RE. Maximal respiratory pressures. Normal values and relationship to age and sex. Am Rev Respir Dis 1971;103:641–650.
6. Braun NMT, Arora NS, Rochester DF. Respiratory muscle and pulmonary function in polymyositis and other proximal myopathies. Thorax 1983;38:616–623.
7. Krowka MJ, Enright PL, Rodarte JR, Hyatt RE. Effect of effort on measurement of forced expiratory volume in one second. Am Rev Respir Dis 1987;16:829–833.
8. Suratt PM, Gal TJ, Hooe DM. Effect of head flexion on airway resistance measured in a body plethysmograph. Br J Dis Chest 1981;75:204–206.
9. Rozas CJ, Goldman AL. Daily spirometric variability. Normal subjects and subjects with chronic bronchitis with and without airflow obstruction. Arch Intern Med 1982;142:1287–1291.
10. Cockroft DW, Berscheld BA. Volume adjustment of maximum mid expiratory flow. Importance of changes in total lung capacity. Chest 1980;78:595–600.
11. Bouhuys A, Hunt VR, Kim BM, Zapletal A. Maximum expiratory flow rates in induced bronchoconstriction in man. J Clin Invest 1969;48:1159–1168.
12. Miller RD, Hyatt RE. Evaluation of obstructing lesions of the trachea and larynx by flow volume loops. Am Rev Respir Dis 1973;108:475–481.
13. Gal TJ, Arora NS. Respiratory mechanics in supine subjects during progressive partial curarization. J Appl Physiol 1982;52:57–63.
14. Vincken WG, Elleker MG, Cusio MG. Flow-volume loop changes reflecting respiratory muscle weakness in chronic neuromuscular disorders. Am J Med 1987;83:673–680.

15. Morris JF, Koski A, Johnson LC. Spirometric standards for healthy non-smoking adults. Am Rev Respir Dis 1971;102:57–67.
16. Clausen JL. Prediction of normal values. In: Clausen JE, ed. Pulmonary function testing guidelines and controversies. Orlando, FL: Grune & Stratton, 1984:49–59.
17. Yakaitas RW, Blitt CD, Angiullo JP. End tidal halothane concentration for endotracheal intubation. Anesthesiology 1977;47:386–388.
18. Pietak S, Weenig CS, Hickey RF, et al. Anesthetic effects on ventilation in patients with chronic obstructive pulmonary disease. Anesthesiology 1975;42:160–166.
19. Connors AF, McAferee D, Gray BA. Effect of inspiratory flow rate on gas exchange during mechanical ventilation. Am Rev Respir Dis 1981;124:537–543.
20. Tuxen DV, Lane S. The effects of ventilatory pattern on hyperinflation, airway pressures, and circulation in mechanical ventilation of patients with severe airflow obstruction. Am Rev Respir Dis 1987;136:872–879.
21. Olsen GN, Block AJ, Swenson EW, et al. Pulmonary function evaluation of the lung resection candidate: a prospective study. Am Rev Respir Dis 1975;111:379–387.
22. Ladurie ML, Ranson Bitker B. Uncertainties in the expected value for forced expiratory volume in one second after surgery. Chest 1986;90:222–228.
23. Smith TP, Kinasewitz GT, Tucker WY, Spillers WP, George RB. Exercise capacity as a predictor of post-thoracotomy morbidity. Am Rev Respir Dis 1984;129:730–734.
24. Stein M, Casara EL. Preoperative pulmonary evaluation and therapy for surgery patients. JAMA 1970;211:787–790.
25. Milledge JS, Nunn JF. Criteria of fitness for anesthesia in patients with chronic obstructive lung disease. Br Med J 1975;3:670–673.
26. Williams CD, Brenowitz JG. "Prohibitive" lung function and major surgical procedures. Am J Surg 1976;132:763–766.
27. Gracey DR, Divertie MB, Didier EP. Preoperative pulmonary preparation of patients with chronic obstructive pulmonary disease. A prospective study. Chest 1979;76:123–129.

Chapter 3

Effects of Anesthetic Drugs and Techniques on Respiratory Mechanics

REGIONAL ANESTHESIA

Most clinicians consider regional anesthetic techniques (spinal, epidural, intercostal block) to be essentially free of clinically significant effects on respiratory mechanics. Some of this opinion stems from the fact that there is no loss of consciousness or airway instrumentation with such techniques. It also relates to the fact that the mechanics of quiet respiration—such as tidal volume and respiratory rate—are not appreciably affected. Indeed, mid or high thoracic levels of motor block have little if any impact on resting ventilation, since the diaphragm is unaffected. Thus it is better able to descend because the abdominal wall, which is relaxed, offers less resistance. There is in essence an increased abdominal compliance. Nevertheless, this same paralysis of abdominal muscles affects forced exhalation. For example, Egbert et al.[1] noted a 50% decrease in the pressure subjects could generate during a forced exhalation after a high spinal block, whereas the ability to generate a negative inspiratory pressure was virtually unimpaired. As a result inspiratory capacity was preserved while expiratory reserve volume decreased. A similar pattern was observed with the motor block associated with epidural anesthesia.[2] Likewise, a milder degree of motor blockade with intercostal block (T6–T12) produced mild decrements in expiratory effort and flow with no effects on inspiratory function.[3]

The limitation of expiratory effort may adversely affect patients with chronic bronchitis, whose ability to generate sufficient pressure for an effective cough may be compromised. This same group of patients with chronic lung disease have demonstrated somewhat confusing changes in pulmonary ventilation after spinal anesthesia in the extreme lithotomy position.[4] Unlike normals who demonstrate reductions in forced vital capacity (FVC) under the

42

same circumstances, these patients did not demonstrate worsening and some showed mild improvement. This has been attributed to an elevation of the diaphragm at end expiration that is assisted by the weight of the abdominal viscera and flexion of the thighs. Similar improvements have been noted with the "emphysema belt," head down, and leaning forward positions.[5, 6] The same effect on the abdominal viscera may adversely affect inspiratory capacity in obese patients, particularly under spinal anesthesia.[7]

GENERAL ANESTHESIA

General anesthesia affects the static (pressure-volume) and the dynamic (pressure-flow) behavior of the respiratory system. These mechanical effects have interested clinicians and investigators because of their potential contribution to the impaired gas exchange characteristic of anesthetized patients. Perhaps no facet of respiratory system behavior has received as much attention as the change in functional residual capacity (FRC). A decrease in FRC with the induction of general anesthesia was first noted by Bergman.[8] Subsequent observations in supine anesthetized humans indicate that FRC is reduced an average of about 500 ml or 15 to 20% of the awake value.[9] The decreased volume is similar in magnitude to that observed when subjects go from erect to recumbent position as noted earlier. The magnitude of FRC reduction appears to be related to age and body habitus (i.e., weight-to-height ratio). In fact, morbidly obese patients demonstrate a much larger decrease in FRC to about 50% of the preanesthetic values.[10]

The changes in FRC occur within a minute after induction of anesthesia,[11] do not appear to progress with time,[12] and are not further affected by the addition of muscle paralysis.[13] A number of factors may contribute to the FRC reduction, but the underlying mechanisms are complex and as yet not totally clear. Some of these possibilities include atelectasis, increased expiratory muscle activity, trapping of gas in distal airways, cephalad displacement of increased lung recoil, and increases in thoracic blood volume.

Atelectasis may contribute to or result from the reduction in FRC. The rapid appearance of densities on computerized tomography supports this possibility.[14] The prompt development of the densities and their lack of dependence on high inspired oxygen concentrations suggest that they may be due to compression of gas, rather than resorption as initially suggested by Dery et al.[15]

Trapping of gas behind closed distal airways does not appear to contribute to the decreased FRC, because measurements of thoracic gas volume have demonstrated the changes in FRC.[16] Furthermore, measurement of nitrogen washout, which measures only gas in contact with the open airways, gave similar results to measurement of total thoracic gas volume by body plethysmography.[13]

During rapid eye movement sleep and with halothane anesthesia the tonic activity of the diaphragm decreases. Muller and associates[17] postulated that this reduced diaphragmatic tone was responsible for the FRC reduction with anesthesia. The intercostal muscles appear to be even more sensitive to depression by volatile agents such as halothane.[18] This would make it attractive to hypothesize that the reduced tone of the diaphragm and intercostals results in a reduced outward recoil of the chest wall. This process does not appear to progress further, since the addition of neuromuscular blockade, which would be expected to diminish muscle tone further, produces no additional changes in FRC. The absence of any additional effect with paralysis also argues against any role of increased tone of the expiratory (abdominal) muscles in determining the end-expiratory lung volume.

Although the changes in FRC could reflect increased elastic recoil of the lungs, most favor the hypothesis that the initial effect is a reduction of outward recoil of the chest wall. The changes in the lung are probably secondary to breathing at low lung volumes. Changes similar to those induced by anesthesia have been demonstrated with chest strapping.[19]

Another possible mechanism contributing to the reduction of FRC may involve a shift of blood from the limbs to the lung and abdomen. The blood in the lungs may have a twofold effect. First, lung congestion may decrease lung compliance and thus increase lung recoil. Second, the blood competes with air for intrathoracic volume. At the same time an increase in abdominal blood volume can act to displace the diaphragm upward or the abdominal wall outward. A report by Hedenstierna et al.[20] suggested that the diaphragm was displaced cranially and that the decrease in the thoracic volume of FRC is associated with a shift of blood from the thorax to the abdomen. Others noted that changes in volume of the rib cage, shape and position of the diaphragm, and intrathoracic fluid (blood) and gas contribute in varying amounts to reducing FRC in different subjects.[21] In the latter study, thoracic gas volume was reduced considerably more than thoracic volume. This suggests that there is some increase in thoracic blood volume with the induction of anesthesia.

Reduction in functional residual capacity with intravenous agents differs from the more dramatic effect of inhalation anesthetics. Thiopental[11] and methohexital[22] produced changes in nonintubated subjects that were similar to those associated with normal sleep.[23] In most cases the decrement in FRC was less than 200 ml. The relatively small magnitude of change was attributed to maintenance of rib cage activity in contrast to the marked depression seen with agents such as halothane.[18] Another intravenous agent, ketamine, also appears to have a sparing action on intercostal muscle activity and is associated with a maintenance of FRC at awake levels in adults[24] and in children.[25] In the latter group the increased respiratory rates and prolonged passive lung emptying as illustrated by the time constant (τ) were associated with an FRC greater than the relaxation volume of the respiratory system (Vrx).[26] The authors speculated that the prolonged lung emptying with ketamine anesthesia was the result of increases in respiratory system compliance (thus τ, the product of

$R \times C$, is increased). With halothane τ is shortened, presumably because respiratory system compliance decreases.

Most changes in the mechanical properties can be ascribed to the smaller size of the respiratory system under anesthesia. The increased lung elastic recoil could reduce FRC but is most likely the result of the reduction of FRC. The data of Westbrook et al.[13] indicate that FRC and compliance are reduced proportionately. This suggests that specific compliance (i.e., compliance related to lung volume) in the awake and anesthetized states are rather similar.

In contrast to the pressure-volume characteristics, the pressure-flow characteristics of the respiratory system have received far less attention. Only several studies have compared measurements of pulmonary resistance (RL) in the awake and anesthetized states. With only one exception[27] most have noted increases in resistance following induction of anesthesia and tracheal intubation.[28–31] There are a number of problems interpreting these changes in RL. One relates to the limitations of estimating pleural pressure from esophageal pressure, while another concerns the measurement of airway pressure at the proximal or mouth end of the tracheal tube and not in the trachea beyond the distal end of the tube. In the latter case transpulmonary pressure, the pressure drop across the lung, may be underestimated, as will the calculated RL. Finally, the substitution of a fixed value of tube resistance calculated in vitro must be questioned since the latter can actually exceed the combined resistance of lungs and tube in situ.[32]

Foremost among the mechanisms that might contribute to changes in pulmonary resistance with induction of general anesthesia are the physical properties of the gas mixture of volatile agent, oxygen, and nitrous oxide, which differ from air and oxygen with respect to density and viscosity. Nitrous oxide is more dense than air or oxygen. Thus resistance to turbulent flow, which is directly related to density, could increase with high concentrations of nitrous oxide in the gas mixture. In contrast, the viscosity of a nitrous oxide–oxygen mixture is less than that of air. Thus resistance to laminar flow might be expected to decrease. These changes are complex and impossible to predict, however, and are unlikely to account for most of the changes in RL seen with anesthesia.

Of greater importance is airway caliber, which in addition to smooth muscle tone may be affected by accumulation of secretions, changes in lung elastic recoil, and, most importantly, lung volume. Airway caliber would be expected to be reduced by general anesthesia solely because of the reduced FRC (see Fig. 1.6). Even in the absence of changes in bronchomotor tone, resistance would be expected to be passively increased by more than one-third. When one factors in the influence of tracheal intubation and airway manipulation and the opposing bronchodilating properties of inhalation anesthetics[33] it is no wonder elucidation of the mechanisms controlling pulmonary resistance in the anesthetized patient has been difficult.

Changes in pulmonary resistance (RL) have usually been thought to represent changes in airway resistance (Raw) and to reflect little of the pulmonary tissue resistance (Rti). The latter depends on the pressure-volume hysteresis of lung tissue as lung volume changes. The Rti fraction has been shown to constitute a significant portion of the decreased RL produced by halothane.[34] These findings indicate that it is not appropriate to interpret changes in RL as having a direct effect on Raw or airway caliber.

MUSCLE RELAXANTS

The use of muscle relaxants has transformed anesthetic practice by allowing safe levels of anesthesia to be used while providing adequate surgical conditions. The initial reports of anesthesia using curare with cyclopropane extolled the drug's freedom from cardiorespiratory effects.[35] This opinion was not shared by the majority of anesthetists who commonly experience respiratory difficulty in curarized patients postoperatively. At this point it was not certain whether these respiratory problems arose purely because of peripheral muscle weakness or because of central actions of the drug—as a depressant or analgesic. This was very nicely clarified in a study by Smith,[36] who underwent curarization while awake and concluded that the drug's effects on respiration were solely due to muscle weakness with no central nervous system effects. He made additional observations that suggest a possible effect on proprioception and airway mechanics.

Shortly thereafter a number of studies appeared that were aimed at finding drugs that produced marked peripheral muscle function (grip strength) and spared respiratory function (vital capacity). The report of Unna and Pelikan[37] is typical of such studies, which attempted to find equipotent doses of relaxant drugs that decrease grip strength by 95% while minimally affecting vital capacity. It initially appeared that depolarizing blockers had much less ability to achieve this "respiratory sparing" action. These studies underscored the difficulty in establishing equipotent doses. Recent work indicates that vital capacity was spared relative to grip strength during careful infusion of succinylcholine.[38]

Assessments of what constitutes normal ventilation in the face of neuromuscular blockade have been performed repeatedly, since restoration of adequate ventilation is of prime concern in the curarized patient. Of even more concern is the patient's ability to maintain airway integrity and cope with factors that might impede gas exchange and ventilation. A recent report has shown that the presence of adequate ventilation during recovery from neuromuscular blockade does not indicate the capability of maintaining functional integrity of the upper airway.[39] To fully grasp the importance of this information it is helpful to consider some of the changes in respiratory mechanics that occur with partial neuromuscular blockade.

Tidal volume (VT) is easily measured but it constitutes only about 10 to

15% of the vital capacity. Thus VT can be quite normal in spite of severely limited respiratory function. This same resting breathing, which appears adequate, may easily be compromised by stresses such as airway obstruction or vomiting. Minute ventilation likewise is of limited value in identifying respiratory muscle weakness, since it can be maintained by a corresponding increase in frequency even if VT decreases. Interestingly enough, breathing patterns in some partially curarized subjects were characterized by an increase in VT and minute ventilation.[40]

Of all the tests of actual ventilatory function, none has been more commonly used to assess muscle weakness than the measurement of vital capacity (VC). The extremes of lung volume are achieved with maximal effort such that decrements in VC would at first seem to be related directly and simply to degrees of respiratory muscle weakness. However, the shape of the normal pressure-volume curve of the relaxed respiratory system suggests that this should not be the case (see Fig. 1.3). The relationship between pressure and volume is curvilinear such that near the extremes of lung volume, large changes in pressure or, if you will, strength and effort should occur before volume begins to decrease significantly. In patients with chronic neuromuscular weakness the decrease in VC does not conform to this prediction, largely because of coexistent pulmonary disease and skeletal deformities.[41] Also, in seated subjects partial curarization produced decrements in VC that somewhat exceeded predictions.[42] In contrast, supine curarized subjects experienced reductions in VC that were proportionately less than decreases in respiratory muscle strength and in agreement with predictions based on respiratory system pressure-volume relationships.[43]

The differing data in seated and supine curarized subjects most likely relates to the greater importance of the contribution of inspiratory capacity (IC) to VC in the supine subject and the relatively greater efficiency of the diaphragm in the supine position. The sitting subjects have a higher FRC. Thus, the expiratory portion of VC (expiratory reserve volume, or ERV) assumes a greater importance. The expiratory muscles in turn are significantly more weakened by d-tubocurarine (DTC) than the inspiratory muscles.

The major inspiratory muscle is the diaphragm. It is the only muscle active during quiet respiration. Both in vitro and in vivo observations suggest that the diaphragm is relatively resistant to curare in doses that abolish head lift and hand grip. Because of this, it has been assumed that the diaphragm is spared. A quantitative index of diaphragm function can be obtained by measuring transdiaphragmatic pressure (Pdi), the pressure developed across the contracting diaphragm. Pressures above and below the diaphragm are recorded with balloon catheters placed in the stomach and esophagus to sense intraabdominal and pleural pressures, respectively.

With curarization to levels that abolish head lift and hand grip, maximum static Pdi was 40% of control at FRC and reduced to similar proportion at other volumes.[44] Thus, at this level of curarization, diaphragmatic strength is markedly impaired. This weakness had no effect on tidal volume and resulted in a moderate decrease in inspiratory capacity, which roughly reflected the reduction in Pdi. During maximum voluntary ventilation (MVV), however, ventilation decreased well before the Pdi generated during the maneuver changed. Only with severe weakness did the Pdi decrease below normal, but the decrease was still strikingly less than the severe reduction in MVV.

At slight degress of paralysis, the reduced MVV may be due to incoordination of other respiratory muscles during the intense effort. They are richly endowed with muscle spindles, and thus proprioception may be impaired. This discoordination has been noted in volunteers immediately following reversal when strength appears normal. At more intense levels of paralysis, two other factors appear to contribute to the decreased MVV. The first is upper airway obstruction and the other is the diminished contribution of the other respiratory muscles (accessories, intercostals, and abdominals). The latter are important at high levels of ventilatory effort but appear to be far more sensitive to neuromuscular blockade than the diaphragm.

During partial paralysis, despite marked expiratory muscle weakness, mid-expiratory flows were well maintained during maximal forced expiration.[45] Inspiratory flows were decreased by decreased inspiratory muscle strength or effort. A further decrease in flow appeared to be due to dynamic inspiratory obstruction, as suggested by the character of the inspiratory flow trace. In others the reduced, flattened inspiratory flow pattern may simply represent impaired abduction of the weakened vocal cords.[46]

Another important and yet seldom studied area is the influence of muscle weakness on cough function. In addition to reducing lung volumes and overall ventilatory capacity, respiratory muscle weakness would be expected to decrease coughing ability. Loss of inspiratory muscle power can limit the inspiratory volume that can be developed. Weakness of the laryngeal adductor muscles can reduce the effectiveness of glottic closure necessary at the end of inspiration to generate high intrathoracic pressures. Finally, paralysis of abdominal and other expiratory muscles limits the driving pressure required to expel air in adequate amounts and at velocities sufficient to remove secretions from the airway.[1] Measurements of cough function have been reported in healthy volunteers during voluntary coughing while curarized to a point of head lift and hand grip abolition.[47] A burst of three coughs was initiated from total lung capacity (TLC) to mimic a bout of repetitive coughing.

Between each cough, the glottis closes, pressure builds up, and flow is interrupted (Fig. 3.1). In the curarized subject (Fig. 3.1, right panel), the driving pressure is reduced markedly, but the glottis appears competent to allow flow to be interrupted between cough bursts. Flow rates at the point of maximum pressure development or effort are not reduced appreciably despite marked reductions in pleural pressure. Actually, they are shifted over the volume axis because of a decreased inspiratory volume prior to coughing. The

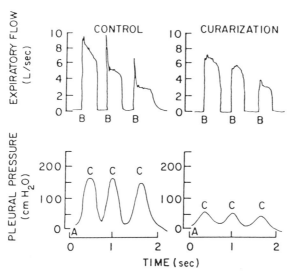

Figure 3.1. Simultaneous records of expiratory flows and pleural pressures during bursts of three successive coughs uninterrupted by inspiration to illustrate changes between control state and weakness with partial curarization. Cough is initiated at total lung capacity. *A*, initial glottic closure; *B*, onset of flow (opening of glottis); *C*, point of maximal driving pressure. (Reproduced with permission from Arora NS, Gal TJ. Cough dynamics during progressive muscle weakness in healthy curarized subjects. J Appl Physiol 1981;51:494–498.)

total volume exhaled during the coughs was reduced by 25%, about the same extent as the decrease in inspiratory capacity. On the surface it appears that cough function is not so much affected by the muscle groups that are more severely weakened (abdominals, intercostals, pharyngeal) but rather by the reduced inspiratory volume. Although decreases in pleural pressure have minimal effect on cough flow rates, compressive airway narrowing—essential for the increased linear velocity and high kinetic energy of effective coughing—is reduced. This is evident in coughs initiated at TLC by the absence of peak flow transients so prominent in the control state (Fig. 3.1).

In surgical patients the postoperative restoration of muscle strength is aimed at providing adequate ventilation; little attention is given to ensuring adequate patency of the upper airway. Pavlin et al.[39] have shown that airway protection may be inadequate when the ability to ventilate per se is deemed adequate by the time-honored criterion of a maximum inspiratory pressure of $(-)25$ cm H_2O. The ability to swallow or to maintain an unobstructed airway was associated with inspiratory pressures of about twice that. The ability to sustain a head lift for 5 seconds was uniformly associated with the ability to provide adequate airway protection. It is important to note that the performance of the head lift must be accomplished with a closed mouth,[48] since the inability to elevate the mandible is highly suggestive of inability to maintain the airway. One must be careful not to allow the presence of an endotracheal tube to obscure this observation.

TRACHEAL INTUBATION

The presence of an endotracheal (ET) tube in the trachea may itself alter respiratory funtion in several ways. First, the ET tube imposes a mechanical burden to breathing since it acts as a fixed inspiratory and expiratory resistor that reduces upper airway caliber. This increased resistance does not appear to be of much significance during quiet breathing[49] but begins to exert a more marked effect during maneuvers requiring greater degrees of effort.[50] Second, the tube bypasses the larnyx and partially splints the trachea, each of which are important determinants of airflow resistance and important components of normal coughing. Finally, mechanical irritation of the larynx and trachea elicits reflexes such as coughing and constriction of airways distal to the tube. This further stimulation of the tracheobronchial tree provokes reflex mucus secretion, which tends to offset the role of the tube in promoting tracheal toilet and may result in additional coughing and bronchoconstriction.[51]

There is little disagreement that an ET tube acts as a fixed inspiratory and expiratory resistor that may represent a burden to the spontaneously breathing patient. However, when the tube is inserted it does not simply add to a patient's normal total airway resistance but rather substitutes for the resistance of the upper airway, i.e., from the mouth to the midtrachea. This portion of the respiratory tract in adults has an average volume of about 72 ml,[52] whereas the internal volume of a standard 8.0-mm I.D. tube is 12 to 15 ml. However, a patient's upper airway volume may vary by as much as 50% with changes in head position.[52] Therefore, the ET tube in some situations may substitute a relatively small but predictable upper airway volume and caliber for a highly unpredictable one.

Pressure-flow relationships of the respiratory system tend to be alinear, largely because of the turbulent flow patterns in the upper airway, especially at the glottis. Major changes in upper airway resistance occur throughout the respiratory cycle and are principally the result of changes in glottic cross-sectional area with movements of the vocal cords. The cross-sectional area of the glottis oscillates around a mean value of 66 mm^2 during quiet breathing,[53] whereas pharyngeal size is almost 10 times that. The cross-sectional area of the trachea is more than 150 mm^2 and may be as high as 300 mm^2.

Attempts to quantitate the actual magnitude of the airflow resistance imposed by ET tubes have largely consisted of assessing the resistance of the tube in isolation. This method, which measures the pressure drop across the tube at a constant flow rate, has been criticized because patients do not breathe with constant flow rates. Instead, flow varies in a sinusoidal fashion during inspiration and expiration. Resistance, which is a function of flow rates, therefore varies likewise. Furthermore, this in vitro measurement of the pressure drop during a constant flow may overestimate the actual resistance of the tube in vivo. The resistance of the tube measured in isolation in many cases actually exceeds the combined resistance of the tube in situ and the remaining respiratory system because of the abrupt change in cross-sectional area between the tube and trachea.[54]

The resistance of a tube depends somewhat on its radius of curvature in situ. In tubes with a smaller radius of curvature, the pressure drop associated with a given flow (i.e., resistance) will be greater than that of a tube whose radius of curvature is larger. The larger tube, because of its smaller pressure drop, produces less resistance to breathing.[55] When inserted in a patient, the bend of a nasotracheal tube has a smaller radius of curvature compared to the same tube inserted orally. Thus an oral tracheal tube offers less resistance to airflow. The oral route also allows for insertion of a shorter tube and one of large internal diameter. The latter is probably the most important variable, since the pressure drop down the tube (and hence resistance) is related inversely to the fourth power for turbulent flow.

The data of Sahn et al.[56] emphasize these differences in resistance between various sizes of ET tubes, which have important clinical implications. With flow rates such as might occur during deep breathing (1 liter/sec), the resistance of a 7.0-mm tube is approximately twice that of an 8.0-mm tube. On the other hand, a 9.0-mm tube produces only about one-third the airflow resistance of an 8.0-mm tube at the very same flow rates. The presence of an ET tube tends to elicit increased secretions, and its accompanying discomfort may limit the depth of inspiration. One could speculate that both factors might result in reduced lung volumes and increased lung stiffness or recoil. Observations in intubated subjects, however, fail to indicate any significant decreases in TLC or lung recoil.[50]

The resting end-expiratory position of the respiratory system, the functional residual capacity (FRC), is the volume at which the inward recoil of the lungs is opposed by an equal outward recoil of the chest wall. In infants, FRC appears to be a "dynamic" balance of forces and occurs at a higher volume than the true static FRC because of the high respiratory rates of infants and possibly because of a high expiratory resistance associated with glottic action. The data of Berman et al.[57] suggest that the presence of an ET tube in infants significantly reduces FRC and impairs oxygenation as a result of interference with glottic action.

Others have similarly hypothesized that the expiratory flow resistance imposed by normal glottic function is also an important determinant of FRC in adults. By excluding this mechanism, an ET tube should impair the ability of the glottis to decrease expiratory flow and to maintain a normal FRC. The data of Annest et al.[58] have been cited as evidence to support this possibility, since their patients exhibited an average FRC decrease of 350 ml while intubated. However, in four of their nine patients, FRC during intubation was virtually identical to that after extubation. On the other hand, in a group of patients with moderate airway obstruction, FRC increased significantly by more than 30% following insertion of an ET tube for fiberoptic bronchoscopy.[59] The absolute magnitude of this FRC increase approached 1 liter in most patients. Such an observation in bronchitic patients is in keeping with what may be expected when peripheral airway constriction occurs and airway resistance is increased. This tends to dispute the relative importance of the expiratory flow resistance from glottic narrowing in determining the normal adult FRC.

The glottic aperture is actually wider during inspiration and indeed narrows during expiration. The cords move toward the midline during expiration to produce a variable controlled resistance, which regulates airflow. This glottic narrowing, however, primarily determines the rate at which the respiratory system returns to its resting volume (FRC) but not the actual volume.[60] Furthermore, this braking of expiratory airflow by vocal cord adduction is reduced during hyperpnea[61] such that one would not expect to hear the audible grunting characteristic of infants. Only during full active expiration to residual volume does the glottic aperture narrow significantly and reach a minimal size at or near residual volume.

In keeping with this, normal healthy subjects intubated after administration of topical anesthesia showed no significant change in FRC measurements (Fig. 3.2).[62] This finding argues against any notion that the glottis plays an important role in determining the FRC in adults as it may in infants. In only two subjects did the changes in FRC exceed normal variations expected with duplicate measurements. One subject showed a decrease of 17%, while FRC increased in another subject by 13%. The latter subject continued to show an increased FRC following extubation, a phenomenon that may have resulted from persistent peripheral airway constriction. In any event, while FRC or end-expiratory volume may be influenced by dynamic factors such as overall airway resistance, it would appear that in normal adults FRC is largely determined by the static balance of forces between the lung and chest wall, and thus is not significantly altered in normals by the presence of an ET tube.

There is abundant physiological information concerning alterations in the pattern of breathing when breathing through external resistances equivalent to endotracheal tubes. In the face of such increased resistance, subjects tend to decrease their respiratory rate while increasing tidal volume in an effort to minimize the work of breathing. Although observations are scant in patients whose tracheas are actually intubated, data on eight postoperative patients[49] and unpublished observations of six normal subjects[62] do not indicate that any significant changes in respiratory rate or tidal volume occur as a result of tracheal intubation.

During normal quiet breathing, peak inspiratory and expiratory flow rates in normal adults are about 0.5 liter/sec or less. During the vigorous expiration associated with a forced vital capacity (FVC) maneuver, flow rates may be 15 to 20 times that. At such flow rates the increased resistance imposed by the ET tube would be expected to affect flows significantly. Indeed, both patients[59] and normals[50] exhibited decreases in 1-second forced expiratory volume (FEV_1) of 20% or more following intubation with 8.0-mm tubes. In normal sub-

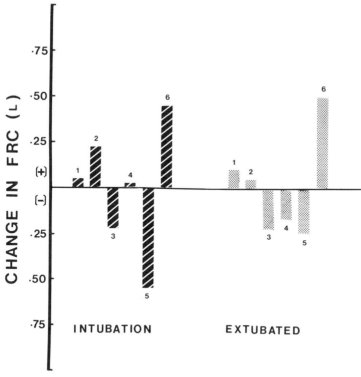

Figure 3.2. Individual changes in FRC compared to control after tracheal intubation and extubation for six healthy subjects. (Reproduced with permission from Gal TJ. How does tracheal intubation alter respiratory mechanics? In: Bishop MJ, ed. Physiology and consequences of tracheal intubation. Philadelphia: JB Lippincott, 1988:2:191–200. Problems in Anesthesia.)

jects FVC was also reduced (12%), whereas the slow vital capacity was not. While the decreased FEV_1 in normal subjects can be accounted for entirely by the tube-imposed resistance, the decrease in FVC in the face of a normal slow VC cannot be explained unless expiratory efforts were submaximal. This was clearly not the case, since expiratory pressure and hence effort were actually increased in the intubated subjects. This discrepancy between slow and forced vital capacity seems to be best explained by the occurrence of air trapping from constriction in airways distal to the ET tube. This phenomenon is also observed when patients with airway obstruction perform forced expirations during pulmonary function testing.

In the presence of many lesions causing upper airway obstruction, inspiratory flow tends to be reduced more than expiratory flow, such that the mid-VC ratio is increased above 1.0. A fixed obstruction such as an external ET tube reduces both inspiratory and expiratory flows equally (Fig. 3.3). Expiratory flow shows a plateau over the initial effort-dependent portion of VC. However, at lower lung volumes near RV where flow is less influenced by maximal effort, flows are about the same as in the control state. With intubation, inspi-

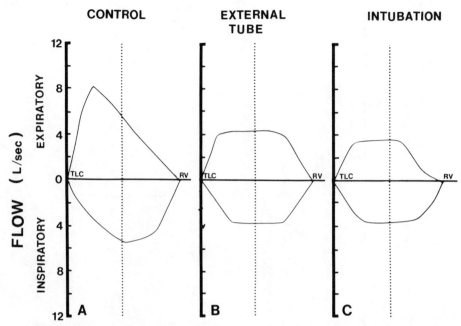

Figure 3.3. Flow-volume loops from a single subject comparing control pattern (**A**) with the effects of the endotracheal tube externally (**B**) and in situ (**C**). The *dotted line* is the midpoint of vital capacity. (Reproduced with permission from Gal TJ. How does tracheal intubation alter respiratory mechanics? In Bishop MJ, ed. Physiology and consequences of tracheal intubation. Philadelphia: JB Lippicott, 1988;2:191–200. Problems in Anesthesia.)

ratory and expiratory flows are reduced similarly at high lung volumes, such that the mid-VC ratio is not significantly changed. However, flow falls below the normal flow-volume envelope at low lung volumes near RV (Fig. 3.3). This decrease in expiratory flow at low lung volumes strongly suggests constriction in airways distal to the tube.

Although airway constriction is most commonly inferred from indices obtained during forced expiration, the measurement of airway resistance (Raw) appears to be the most sensitive and direct technique to identify airway obstruction. The upper limit of normal for Raw is considered to be 2.0 cm H_2O/liter/sec. However, in most healthy, normal subjects it is closer to 1.0 cm H_2O/liter/sec (Fig. 3.4). Such healthy subjects exhibited increases in Raw ranging from 1.2 to 1.5 cm H_2O/liter/sec (mean 1.34) when breathing through 8.0-mm tubes held externally.[62] With the tubes actually in place in the trachea, Raw increased even more. The mean increase above control was 1.75 cm H_2O/liter/sec, resulting in an actual mean Raw value of 2.75. If one accepts the increase in Raw with the external tube as an estimate of tube resistance (1.35), the resistance of the airways distal to the tube can also be estimated at 2.75 − 1.35 = 1.40. In the intubated subjects, the ET tube bypasses the upper airways to the midtrachea. This segment of the airways accounts for

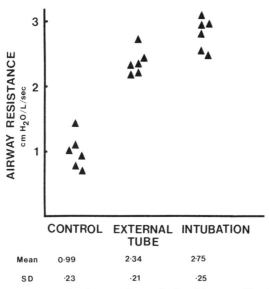

	CONTROL	EXTERNAL TUBE	INTUBATION
Mean	0·99	2·34	2·75
S D	·23	·21	·25

Figure 3.4. Individual changes in airway resistance in six subjects resulting from endotracheal tube externally and in situ. (Reproduced with permission from Gal TJ. How does tracheal intubation alter respiratory mechanics? In: Bishop MD, ed. Physiology and consequences of tracheal intubation. Philadelphia: JB Lippincott, 1988;2:191–200. Problems in Anesthesia.)

about one-third of Raw during mouth breathing,[63] or about 0.33 cm $H_2O/$ liter/sec in the normal volunteers. The Raw in airways distal to the tube would then be about 0.67 cm H_2O/liter/sec. Thus the estimate of 1.40 cm H_2O/liter/ sec in the intubated subjects suggests at least a doubling of resistance in airways distal to the tube. The most likely cause of this dramatic increase in resistance is reflex airway constriction resulting from irritation by the ET tube. Furthermore, since such responses occurred in subjects whose airways were substantially anesthetized by topical local anesthetic, it is reasonable to speculate that airway response would be exaggerated in patients whose tracheas are not anesthetized with topical anesthesia or those in whom adequate depths of general anesthesia have not been established.

During the act of normal coughing, a forceful, sudden expulsion of air occurs. This blast of airflow serves to clear intrapulmonary airways down to the level of the medium-sized bronchi. The effectiveness of coughing in clearing airways depends primarily on the linear velocity of gas in the airway. The latter is a function of high flow and a reduced airway cross-sectional area. Such dramatic narrowing of the airway lumen can be readily observed bronchoscopically during coughing. Measurements indicate that the cross-sectional area of the trachea decreases to as small as 10% of its normal size during a cough.[64] Prior to each cough, contraction of the expiratory muscles produces an increase in airway pressure well above atmospheric pressure. This driving pressure for coughing is normally developed in the presence of a closed glottis.

The presence of an endotracheal tube might be expected to have significant effects on normal coughing. For one thing, the fixed tube resistance is likely to limit expiratory flow rates. Second, the tube eliminates the contribution of the glottis and its sphincteric action during the initial buildup of driving pressure prior to a cough. Finally, the noncollapsible tube functions as a splint and prevents the near obliteration of the tracheal lumen by the collapsing posterior membranous wall.

Cough dynamics were studied in a group of healthy subjects before and after intubation.[65] The bursts of cough resembled a series of forced expirations at decreasing lung volumes (Fig. 3.5), each interrupted by closure of the glottis. Although quantitative conclusions about the effects of the tube are not possible, the study affords some qualitative insight into cough dynamics with an ET tube in place.

In the normal control state, glottic closure occurs (*A* in Fig. 3.5) following a deep inspiration. This allows driving pressure to increase as the expiratory muscles contract. Just before pressure reaches a maximum (*C*), the glottis opens and allows a burst of flow to begin (*B*). Each subsequent cough burst proceeds in the same fashion, but at a decreasing lung volume. With an endotracheal tube in place, glottic closure is eliminated and flow begins early (*B*) while pressure is increasing and reaches its maximum at the same time as max-

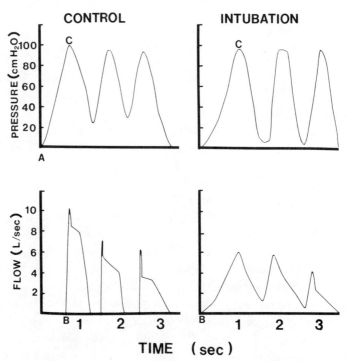

Figure 3.5. A typical burst of three successive coughs measured in healthy subjects before and after tracheal intubation. (Reproduced with permission from Gal TJ. How does tracheal intubation alter respiratory mechanics? In: Bishop MJ, ed. Physiology and consequences of tracheal intubation. Philadelphia: JB Lippincott, 1988;2:191–200. Problems in Anesthesia.)

imal pressure development (*C*). Note also that flow is not entirely interrupted between cough bursts, because glottic action is bypassed. However, the elimination of glottic closure by the tube does not appear to influence the ability to develop high driving pressures during coughing. Instead, the presence of the tube alters the normal timing of pressure and flow such that a cough more closely resembles a normal forced expiration. The resistance of the tube does not allow maximal flows to be reached at high lung volumes in spite of increased effort. At low lung volumes, this increased effort produces compressive narrowing of the large airway distal to the tube. This compression can, by means of a tussive squeeze, transport secretions to the area of the trachea. However, the noncollapsible endotracheal tube tends to maintain the tracheal lumen size, rather than allowing it to collapse. As a result, high flow rates are needed to achieve the linear velocities necessary to clear secretions through this portion of the airways. Secretions, therefore, are likely to accumulate at the area around the end of the tube unless subsequent coughs can be initiated at high lung volume to achieve the high flows possible. Also, since the noncollapsible tube does not permit high velocities, it would appear that optimal tussive efficiency during tracheal intubation would require the shortest possible tube to minimize resistance, and that the tube should be inserted the least possible safe distance below the vocal cords to permit a longer segment of trachea to undergo compressive narrowing.

PHARMACOLOGICAL MODIFICATION OF AIRWAY REACTIVITY DURING ANESTHESIA

Patients with obstructive airway disease such as asthma and chronic bronchitis exhibit exaggerated bronchoconstriction when exposed to a variety of stimuli during the course of anesthesia. The most notable of these of course is airway instrumentation. The heightened bronchial reactivity characteristic of patients with obstructive airway disease has been attributed to a variety of factors, among which are a reduced resting airway caliber, hypertrophy of airway smooth muscle, and increased accessibility of the stimuli to the subepithelial receptors.

Within the airway wall there are three types of sensory receptors whose activity alters bronchial smooth muscle tone, principally via parasympathetic pathways. The slowly adapting pulmonary stretch receptors are abundant deep within the smooth muscle of the posterior tracheal wall but are also found in the walls of the bronchi and small airways. These receptors regulate the rate and depth of breathing and are responsible for the classic Hering-Breuer inflation reflex. Another group, the rapidly adapting irritant receptors, are found throughout the mucosa of all the cartilaginous airways but are most prominent in the trachea and especially at the carina. They respond to mechanical irritation, thermal stimuli, and irritants such as inhaled particles or gases. Airway edema and histamine release also elicit their activity, which results in reflex cough, bronchoconstriction, and mucus secretion. A final group of receptors, the juxtapulmonary ("J") receptors, lie adjacent to pulmonary capillaries in the interstitium between alveoli. They appear to respond to pulmonary congestion, edema, inflammation, and exercise. They play a prominent role in producing the unpleasant sensation of dyspnea that accompanies states such as pulmonary congestion.

PATHOPHYSIOLOGY OF BRONCHOSPASM

Many diverse factors contribute to the development of bronchospasm. In children with asthma, bronchospasm usually develops during exposure to allergens, or from the edema and inflammation associated with viral infections. Treatment regimens, therefore, consist primarily of mediator inhibitors and anti-inflammatory drugs. In adults with airway obstruction allergy is far less important. Irritant-induced bronchoconstriction provides the most significant problem in the anesthetic management of these patients. Tracheal intubation, for example, is a potent irritating stimulus, especially if some bronchocarinal stimulation occurs. It is therefore important to understand the pathways involved in this parasympathetic reflex arc (Fig. 3.6), as well as the multiple sites at which the reflex can be interrupted pharmacologically. In most cases the compounds that interrupt the reflex arc are more effective in preventing than reversing preexisting bronchospasm.

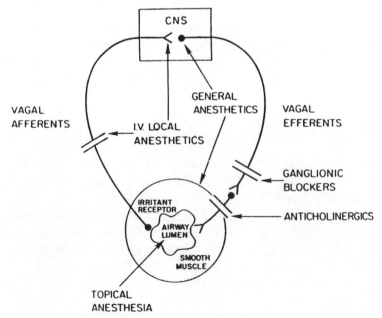

Figure 3.6. Parasympathetic reflex pathways involved in airway constriction indicate the multiple sites that can be affected by pharmacological agents available to anesthesiologists.

SPECIFIC BRONCHODILATOR DRUGS

β-Adrenergic Agents

The airway smooth muscle, which extends from the trachea to the alveolar ducts, is under the influence of the autonomic nervous system. Parasympathetic innervation via the vagus nerves extends down to the terminal bronchioles and has been demonstrated histologically. There is little evidence for direct innervation of bronchial smooth muscle by the sympathetic nervous system. Despite this, adrenergic agonist drugs have enjoyed much more widespread use in managing bronchospasm compared to cholinergic antagonist compounds.

Epinephrine, a natural catecholamine, has been used for many years and is the prototype for all sympathomimetics. It is still regarded as the initial therapy in young asthmatics as 0.1 to 0.5-ml subcutaneous doses of the 0.1%. (1:1000) solution. Isoproterenol, another potent β-agonist drug, is usually administered as an aerosol. Responses to both these compounds are mediated via β_1 and β_2 receptors. Thus the desirable β_2 effect of bronchodilation is often accompanied by adverse β_1 effects of cardiac stimulation, in particular tachyarrhythmias.

Newer substituted catecholamines have been developed to provide more β_2 selectivity and a long duration of action. The most notable among these compounds are albuterol, terbutaline, and bitolterol. Currently the most popular β_2-selective drug appears to be albuterol, which is available as a metered-dose inhaler producing about 100 μg per puff (the usual dose is 2 to 4 puffs). Although an I.V. preparation of albuterol is available, its therapeutic usefulness is doubtful. When given by intravenous injection, the initial plasma concentrations can be high enough to effectively abolish β_2 selectivity so that bronchodilation and tachycardia occur to the same degree.[66]

Anticholinergic Agents

The anticholinergics, or more precisely the antimuscarinic compounds, have been used to treat asthma for centuries. They have been largely neglected because of the troublesome systemic side effects associated with atropine. The quaternary ammonium congeners of atropine are poorly absorbed across biological membranes. As aerosols, they produce significant prolonged bronchodilation that is relatively free of side effects.[67] Such agents offer an alternative or complementary therapy for airway obstruction, especially in patients who experience tremor and tachycardia with β-adrenergic drugs and whose bronchodilator response is incomplete despite optimum therapy. Presently, only ipratropium bromide is available as an aerosol and only in a very low-dosage formulation.

Glycopyrrolate, a compound familiar to anesthesiologists, produces bronchodilation of significantly longer duration than atropine when injected intravenously in doses of 1.0 mg.[68] Such large doses of anticholinergics are relatively slow in onset compared to the sympathomimetics, whether given by inhalation or parenteral administration. Thus, these compounds tend to be more effective as prophylaxis than as treatment for active bronchospasm. Such prophylaxis can be readily achieved by I.V. administration prior to induction of anesthesia.

One longstanding area of concern with the use of anticholinergics arises from their actions in reducing secretions. Such therapy was believed to render respiratory secretions more viscid and apt to occlude airways. Concerns about altering the viscosity of secretions and causing inspissation are not supported by existing data, which indicate that these drugs alter the volume of secretions but not their chemical composition.[69]

Methylxanthines

The bronchodilator effect of theophylline is believed to result from inhibition of the enzyme phosphodiesterase, thereby reducing degradation of cyclic adenosine monophosphate (AMP). However, theophylline concentrations that increase cellular levels of cyclic AMP are many times those that produce smooth muscle relaxation and bronchodilation. Other speculations about the action of theophylline include adenosine antagonism,[70] whereas data on subjects with normal airways[71] and on dogs[72] anesthetized with thiopental and fentanyl suggest that bronchodilation with theophyllines occurs largely as a result of catecholamine release and is abolished by β-adrenergic blockade.

The use of aminophylline, the ethylenediamine salt of theophylline, is considered the standard maintenance therapy for bronchospasm despite its rather narrow therapeutic range. On a molar basis it is twice as potent as caffeine, though no more effective.[73] The role of aminophylline in treating or preventing bronchospasm that is likely to be associated with anesthesia is controversial. The potential for arrhythmias and the lack of objective efficacy data, particularly in the presence of halothane,[72] have led to questions about its perioperative use. The routine recommendation for primary therapy of acute bronchospasm in the emergency room has also been questioned seriously.[74]

Corticosteroids

Although their mechanism of action remains unclear, parenteral steroids are important in the preoperative preparation of patients with reactive airway disease and the treatment of intraoperative bronchospasm. Dosage equivalents of 1 to 2 mg/kg hydrocortisone are recommended for good clinical response. In steroid-treated patients these are doubled, since lower plasma corticoid levels result from comparable doses.[75] Preoperative steroid administration is important because their beneficial effects develop slowly. These effects appear largely to be an enhancement of the actions of β-adrenergic drug therapy.[76]

ANESTHETIC DRUGS

Intravenous Induction Agents

Usual clinical induction doses of thiopental leave airway reflexes largely intact and may be associated with bronchospasm if instrumentation of the airway occurs prior to establishing adequate anesthesia. The early observations of Schnider and Papper[77] indicate that thiopental per se is not the cause of bronchospasm and is therefore not contraindicated to induce anesthesia in patients with airway disease. Ketamine has been suggested as the induction agent of choice for patients with bronchospastic disease, especially if a rapid induction is necessary.[78] Ketamine has been shown to cause bronchial smooth muscle relaxation in vitro[79] and to be as effective as enflurane and halothane in preventing mediator-induced bronchospasm in dogs.[80] The latter appears to be related to sympathomimetic properties of ketamine since the protective effect is abolished by β blockade. Clinical data identifying bronchodilating actions of ketamine in humans are scant and largely subjective. One study did provide measurements of total respiratory resistance, but results are obscured by the administration of muscle relaxants following control measurements.[81] Nevertheless, the fact that none of the patients experienced a worsening of bronchospasm supports the notion that ketmaine may well be a useful induction agent in the bronchospastic patient.

Narcotic Analgesics

The use of narcotic analgesics in patients with chronic airway obstruction is controversial because of their well-known inhibition of the respiratory responses to both hypoxia and hypercapnia.[82] Opioids are known to alter the activity of various other neural pathways, including the human cough reflex. Morphine administration has been shown to actually inhibit vagally mediated bronchoconstriction in patients with mild asthma.[83] Although no objective data are available, it is likely that large doses of narcotics will block airway reflexes in a fashion similar to their suppression of cardiovascular reflexes. Because such large doses of morphine are associated with increases in plasma histamine,[84] there has been much concern about the potential effects on airway function. However, histamine injections resulting in much higher blood levels have produced only small, short-lived increases in airway resistance.[85] Furthermore, other more effective opioids such as fentanyl and sufentanil are available for use in high doses to supplement anesthesia. The latter drugs do not appear to be associated with significant histamine release.

Inhalation Anesthetics

Inhalation of anesthetic concentrations of halothane produces bronchodilation. Although this action was originally attributed entirely to the augmentation of β-adrenergic responses,[86] more recent evidence indicates the importance of the depression of airway reflexes and the direct relaxation of airway smooth muscle.[87] Halothane has been considered the agent of choice for the patient with bronchospastic disease; however, its myocardial depressant action and arrhythmic effects in the presence of circulating catecholamines prevent it from being the ideal agent. Both enflurane[88] and isoflurane[87] are equally effective in preventing and reversing bronchoconstriction when significant levels of anesthesia (1.5 MAC) are present. Such anesthetic depth may be difficult to establish prior to tracheal intubation in patients with airway disease because of their marked ventilation-perfusion mismatch and impaired uptake of anesthetic agents.

Local Anesthetics

Lidocaine has been reported as a treatment for intraoperative bronchospasm.[89] Intravenous lidocaine administered to produce clinically useful blood concentrations (1 to 2 μg/ml) prevents reflex bronchoconstriction.[90] Aerosol therapy offers no advantage over the intravenous route and may provoke bronchospasm in susceptible individuals because of airway irritation. In debilitated patients with chronic airway obstruction, infusions of lidocaine (2 to 3 mg/min) may also be useful to reduce anesthetic requirements and minimize airway reactivity if suppression of airway reflexes with inhalation anesthetics cannot be achieved without profound cardiovascular depression.

Neuromuscular Blockers

The administration of d-tubocurarine is associated with release of histamine, a potential bronchoconstrictor. No changes in respiratory resistance were noted in normals receiving curare,[91] but marked increases occurred in patients with preexisting airway obstruction.[92] Since patients with similar elevated respiratory resistance did not show increases with pancuronium, the authors concluded that changes were likely to be a result of sensitivity to histamine. Since vagal reflexes play a role in the mechanisms of histamine-induced bronchospasm, vagal blockade with anticholinergics may provide some protection.[93, 94]

A factor of equal importance concerns the need to reverse the actions of nondepolarizing blockers. In patients with airway obstruction the muscarinic actions of cholinesterase inhibitors such as neostigmine may increase airway secretions and precipitate bronchospasm. It appears prudent to administer larger than customary doses of glycopyrrolate (more than 0.5 mg) or atropine (more than 1.0 mg) to minimize this possibility when reversal is required. An alternate approach would entail the use of short-acting relaxants to allow their effects to wear off sufficiently to require reversal for airway protection.

DIAGNOSIS AND THERAPY OF INTRAOPERATIVE BRONCHOSPASM

Episodes of wheezing during anesthesia are not uncommon and may result from phenomena other than simple reactive bronchospasm. Such causes of nonasthmatic wheezing must be considered prior to initiating definitive treatment of bronchospasm. Endobronchial intubation, for example, may result in dramatic increases in airway pressure during mechanical ventilation, since gas delivery is confined to one lung. The presence of the tube at the carina may also stimulate the very abundant and sensitive irritant receptors in this area and actually produce reflex bronchospasm. More commonly, such irritation is manifested by persistent coughing and straining, which require the use of high inflation pressures. The use of muscle relaxants to differentiate this from actual bronchoconstriction has been emphasized.[95] Excessive lung inflation pressures may also result from mechanical obstruction of the endotracheal tube from kinking, inspissated secretions, or overinflation of the cuff. Usually such obstruction is associated with audible noises throughout both inspiratory and expiratory phases of respiration. Diagnosis may be inferred by failed attempts to pass a suction catheter but may be verified only with fiberoptic bronchoscopy.

Several mechanical ventilators still available for anesthetic use employ a bellows that ascends during inspiration and descends during expiration. The rapid descent of such bellows produces subambient pressures within the anesthetic circuit and accelerates expiratory flow in a manner comparable to that in the presence of mild expiratory effort. The result is a wheeze-like sound during the final portion of expiration. The sounds originate not because of active airway constriction but rather because the airways undergo dynamic collapse as they reach flow limitation.

Early in the development of pulmonary edema interstitial fluid has been noted to accumulate around bronchioles in a cuff-like fashion. This phenomenon is believed to be responsible for the increased airway resistance associated with pulmonary congestion and results in wheezing that is most prominent near the end of exhalation. Cooperman and Price[96] noted that this wheezing was a prominent early sign in surgical patients who developed pulmonary edema in the operative and postoperative periods. Obviously, effective treatment in these patients must be directed at correcting the cardiac failure rather than producing bronchodilation.

Another condition that may present with clinical signs similar to actual bronchospasm is tension pneumothorax. Recognition of pneumothorax is often delayed because of the similarity of presentation and also because many of the patients in whom pneumothoraces occur have chronic obstructive airway disease.[97] Presumably the wheezing originates because of bronchiolar compression associated with the reduced volume of the affected lung. Hypotension and tachycardia are early signs of pneumothorax that may help in distinguishing it from true bronchospasm; however, definitive diagnosis and treatment may be confirmed only by demonstrating gas escape through a large-bore needle inserted anteriorly into the second intercostal space.

Aspiration of gastric contents into the tracheobronchial tree must also be considered as a cause of bronchospasm, although it is less likely to occur in patients whose tracheas are intubated. The aspiration of gastric contents stimulates irritant receptors and results in constriction of the major airways. In most cases airway constriction is self-limited, and efforts should be devoted to correcting gas exchange abnormalities. A similar therapeutic approach is appropriate for pulmonary embolism. Wheezing in the latter is believed to be related to the release of bronchoconstrictive amines into the peripheral airways. There is some dispute, however, concerning the actual importance of wheezing as a major finding in pulmonary embolism.[98]

When the diagnosis of bronchospasm is established during the use of a general anesthetic, the initial therapy may consist simply of increasing the depth of anesthesia. The use of profound levels of inhalation anesthesia may not be totally effective in severe bronchospasm and may produce severe hypotension and arrhythmias.[99] Despite these cardiovascular limitations, anecdotal reports continue to tout the use of deep inhalation anesthesia to treat status asthmaticus.[100, 101]

In anesthetized patients who are not already paralyzed, skeletal muscle relaxation is essential since vigorous expiratory efforts may worsen airway obstruction. Paralysis also helps to determine whether the increased airway pressures and difficulty in ventilating are due to actual bronchospasm or merely straining and coughing on the endotracheal tube.

The decreased airway caliber associated with bronchoconstriction profoundly affects the distribution of gases within the lung. The major effect is underventilation of many lung units. The net result of this maldistribution of ventilation relative to perfusion is arterial hypoxemia. The pulmonary vasodilating properties of many bronchodilating agents further worsen these ventilation-perfusion relationships. Thus it is important in the anesthetized patient to increase the inspired oxygen concentration as high as possible in the presence of bronchospasm.

The mechanical ventilation of patients who develop airflow obstruction has been controversial. Some have recommended low inspiratory flow rates to minimize peak airway pressures[102] and to improve the distribution of ventilation to obstructed areas.[103] Others have emphasized the need for high inspiratory flow rates to maximize the expiratory time necessary for emptying of obstructed airways. Evidence in two recent studies clearly supports this latter recommendation.[104, 105] Increased inspiratory flows reduced pulmonary hyperinflation, improved gas exchange, and lessened circulatory depression. The peak pressures in these patients increased with increased flows, but a large component was expended on the resistance of the breathing system and tracheal tube and thus was not reflected in alveolar pressure.

Therapy with intravenous lidocaine (2 mg/kg) and atropine (1 to 2 mg) or glycopyrrolate (1 mg) may be helpful in reversing some of the bronchoconstriction, but such agents are far more valuable as prophylaxis. Similarly, the use of corticosteroids (hydrocortisone 4 mg/kg) is also more appropriate as prophylaxis because of delays in the onset of action. The cornerstone of the treatment of intraoperative bronchospasm is inhalation of sympathomimetics such as albuterol. These agents can be administered conveniently to the anesthetic circuit (Fig. 3.7) and produce rapid and effective bronchodilation, although delivery of such agents is less efficient than in the spontaneously breathing patient.[106]

Recommended therapy for intraoperative bronchospasm has always included intravenous aminophylline (5 mg/kg over 10 minutes and 0.9 mg/kg/hr). In patients already receiving theophyllines, acute administration intraoperatively may result in blood levels approaching toxic ranges and the increased likelihood of cardiac arrhythmias when given with halothane. The potential interaction of aminophylline with the sympathomimetics must also be considered. The use of aminophylline in the anesthetized patient remains

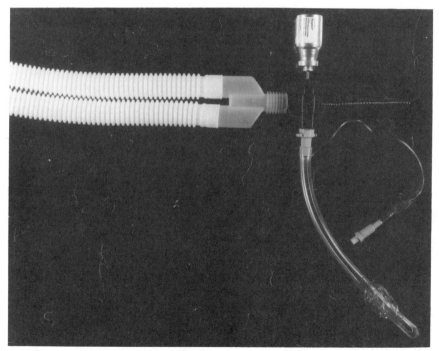

Figure 3.7.   An elbow adapter for placement between the anesthetic circuit and the endotracheal tube. Removal of the cap allows placement of an aerosol canister and administration of medication directly down the tube. (Bronchodilator tee, Boehringer Laboratories, Inc. Wynnewood, PA.)

controversial not only because of cardiotoxicity and arrhythmias but also because of continuing questions regarding its efficacy.[107]

REFERENCES

1. Egbert LD, Tamersoy K, Deas TC. Pulmonary function during spinal anesthesia: the mechanism of cough depression. Anesthesiology 1961;22:882–885.
2. Freund FG, Bonica JJ, Ward RJ, Akamatsu TJ, Kennedy WF. Ventilatory reserve and level of motor block during high spinal and epidural anesthesia. Anesthesiology 1967;28:834–837.
3. Hecker BR, Bjurstrom R, Schoene RB. Effect of intercostal nerve blockade on respiratory mechanics and CO_2 chemosensitivity at rest and exercise. Anesthesiology 1989;70:13–18.
4. Glesecke AH, Cale JO, Jenkins MT. The prostate ventilation and anesthesia. JAMA 1968;203:389–391.
5. Barach AL, Beck GJ. Ventilatory effects of head down position in pulmonary emphysema. Am J Med 1954;16:55–60.
6. Barach AL. Chronic obstructive lung disease: postural relief of dyspnea. Arch Phys Med Rehabil 1974;55:494–504.
7. Catenacci AJ, Sampathacar KR. Ventilatory studies in the obese paitent during spinal anesthesia. Anesth Analg 1969;48:48–54.
8. Bergman NA. Distribution of inspired gas during anesthesia and artificial ventilation. J Appl Physiol 1963;18:1085–1089.
9. Rehder K, Marsh HM. Respiratory mechanics during anesthesia and mechanical ventilation. In: Macklem PT, Mead J, eds. Handbook of physiology. The respiratory system. Mechanics of breathing. Bethesda, MD: American Physiological Society 1986;737–752.
10. Damia G, Mascheroni D, Croci M, Tarenzi L. Perioperative changes in functional residual capacity in morbidly obese patients. Br J Anaesth 1988;60:574–578.
11. Bergman NA. Reduction in resting end-expiratory position of the respiratory system with induction of anesthesia and neuromuscular paralysis. Anesthesiology 1982;57:1417.
12. Hewlett AM, Hulands GH, Nunn JF, Milledge JS. Functional residual capacity during anesthesia. II. Spontaneous respiration. Br J Anaesth 1974;46:486–494.
13. Westbrook PR, Stubbs SE, Sessler AD, Rehder K, Hyatt RE. Effects of anesthesia and muscle paralysis on respiratory mechanics in normal man. J Appl Physiol 1973;34:81–86.
14. Brismar B, Hedenstierna G, Lundquist H, Strandberg A, Svensson L, Tokics L. Pulmonary densities during anesthesia with muscular relaxation—a proposal of atelectasis. Anesthesiology 1985;62:422–428.
15. Dery R, Pelletier J, Jaques A, Clavet M, Houde J. Alveolar collapse induced by nitrogenation. Can Anaesth Soc J 1965;12:531–544.
16. Hedenstierna G, Lofstrom B, Lundh R. Thoracic gas volume and chest abdomen dimensions during anesthesia and muscle paralysis. Anesthesiology 1981;55:499–506.
17. Muller N, Volgyesi G, Becker L, Bryan MH, Bryan AC. Diaphragmatic muscle tone. J Appl Physiol 1979;47:279–284.
18. Tusiewicz K, Bryan AC, Froese AB. Contributions of changing rib cage–diaphragm interactions to the ventilatory depression of halothane anesthesia. Anesthesiology 1977;47:327–337.
19. Scheidt M, Hyatt RE, Rehder K. Effect of rib cage or abdominal restriction on lung mechanics. J Appl Physiol 1981;51:1115–1121.
20. Hedenstierna G, Strandberg A, Brismar B, Lundquist H, Svensson L, Tokics L. Functional residual capacity, thoracoabdominal dimensions, and central blood volume during general anesthesia with muscle paralysis and mechanical ventilation. Anesthesiology 1985;62:247–254.
21. Krayer S, Rehder K, Beck KC, Cameron PD, Didier EP, Hoffman EA. Quantification of thoracic volumes by three dimensional imaging. J Appl Physiol 1987;62:591–598.
22. Bickler PE, Dueck R, Prutow R. Effects of barbiturate anesthesia on functional residual

capacity and rib cage/diaphragm contributions to ventilation. Anesthesiology 1987;60:147–182.

23. Hudgel DW, Devadatta P. Decrease in functional residual capacity during sleep in normal humans. J Appl Physiol 1984;57:1319–1322.

24. Mankikian B, Cantineau JP, Sartene R, Clergue F, Viars P. Ventilatory pattern and chest wall mechanics during ketamine anesthesia in humans. Anesthesiology 1986;65:492–499.

25. Shulman D, Bearsmore CS, Aronson HG, Bodfrey S. The effect of ketamine on functional residual capacity in young children. Anesthesiology 1985;62:551–556.

26. Shulman D, Bar-yishay E, Beardsmore C, Godfrey S. Determinants of end-expiratory lung volume in young children during ketamine or halothane anesthesia. Anesthesia 1987;66:636–640.

27. Gold MI, Han YH, Helrich M. Pulmonary mechanics during anesthesia. III. Influence of intermittent positive pressure and relation to blood gases. Anesth Analg 1966:631–641.

28. Wu N, Miller WF, Luhn R. Studies of breathing in anesthesia. Anesthesiology 1956;17:696–707.

29. Rehder K, Mallow JE, Fibuch EE, Krabill DR, Sessler AD. Effects of isoflurane anesthesia and muscle paralysis on respiratory mechanics in normal man. Anesthesiology 1974;41:477–485.

30. Hedenstierna G, McCarthy G. Mechanics of breathing, gas distribution, and functional residual capacity at different frequences of respiration during spontaneous and artificial ventilation. Br J Anaesth 1975;57:706–712.

31. Dohi S, Gold MI. Pulmonary mechanics druing general anesthesia. The influence of mechanical irritation on the airway. Br J Anaesth 1979;51:205–213.

32. Loring SH, Elliott EA, Drazen JM. Kinetic energy loss and convective acceleration in respiratory resistance measurements. Lung 1979;156:33–42.

33. Lehane JR, Jordan C, Jones JG. Influence of halothane and enflurane on respiratory airflow resistance and specific conductance in anesthetized man. Br J Anaesth 1980;52:773–781.

34. Warner DO, Vetterman N, Brusaco V, Rehder K. Pulmonary resistance during halothane anesthesia is not determined only by airway caliber. Anesthesiology 1989;70:453–460.

35. Grifith HR, Johnson GC. The use of curare in general anesthesia. Anesthesiology 1942;3:418–420.

36. Smith SM, Brown HO, Toman JEP, Goodman LS. The lack of cerebral effects of d-tubocurarine. Anesthesiology 1947;8:1–13.

37. Unna KR, Pelikan EW. Evaluation of curarizing drugs in man. VI. critique of experiments on unanesthetized subjects. Ann NY Acad Sci 1951;54:480–489.

38. Williams JP, Bourke DL. Effects of succinylcholine on respiratory and non-respiratory muscle strength in humans. Anesthesiology 1985;63:299–303.

39. Pavlin EG, Holle RH, Schoene RB. Recovery of airway protection compared with ventilation in humans after paralysis with curare. Anesthesiology 1989;70:381–385.

40. Rosenbaum SH, Askanazi J, Hyman AI, Kinney JM. Breathing patterns during curare-induced muscle weakness. Anesth Analg 1983;62:809–814.

41. Detroyer A, Borenstein S, Cordier R. Analysis of lung volume restriction in patients with respiratory muscle weakness. Thorax 1980;35:603–610.

42. Saunders NA, Rigg JRA, Pengelly LD, Campbell EJM. Effect of curare on maximum static P-V relationships of the respiratory system. J Appl Physiol 1978;44:589–595.

43. Gal TJ, Goldberg SK. Relationship between respiratory muscle strength and vital capacity during partial curarization in awake subjects. Anesthesiology 1981;54:141–147.

44. Gal TJ, Goldberg SK. Diaphragmatic function in healthy subjects during partial curarization. J Appl Physiol 1980;48:921–926.

45. Gal TJ, Arora NS. Respiratory mechanics in supine subjects during partial curarization. J Appl Physiol 1982;53:57–63.

46. Bruce DL, Downs JB, Kilkatrnii PS, Capal LM. Precurarization inhibits maximum ventilatory effort. Anesthesiology 1984;61:618–621.

47. Arora NS, Gal TJ. Cough dynamics during progressive muscle weakness in healthy curarized subjects. J Appl Physiol 1981;51:494–498.

48. Kallos T. Open mouthed head lifting, a sign of incompete reversal of neuromuscular blockade. Anesthesiology 1972;37:650–651.

49. Colgan FA, Liang JQ, Barrow RE. Noninvasive assessment by capacitance respirometry of respiration before and after extubation. Anesth Analg 1975;54:807–813.

50. Gal TJ. Pulmonary mechanics in normal subjects following endotracheal intubation. Anesthesiology 1980;52:27–35.

51. Widicombe JG. Mechanism of cough and its regulation. Eur J Respir Dis 1980;61(supl 110):11–15.

52. Nunn JF, Campbell EJM, Peckett B. Anatomical subdivision of the volume of respiratory dead space and effects of positions of the jaw. J Appl Physiol 1959;14:174–176.

53. Baier H, Wanner A, Zarzecki S, Sackner M. Relationships among glottis opening, respiratory flow, and upper airway resistance in humans. J Appl Physiol 1977;43:603–611.

54. Chang HK, Mortola JP. Fluid dynamic factors in tracheal pressure measurements. J Appl Physiol 1981;51:218–225.

55. Habib MP. Physiological implications of artificial airways. Chest 1989;96:180–184.

56. Sahn SA. Laksminarayan S, Petty TI. Weaning from mechanical ventilation. JAMA 1976;235:2208–2212.

57. Berman LS, Fox WW, Raphaely R. Optimum levels of CPAP for tracheal extubation of newborn infants. J Pediatr 1976;89:109–112.

58. Annest SJ, Gottlieb M, Paloski WH, Stratton H, Newell JC, Dutton R, Powers S. Detrimental effects of removing end-expiratory pressure prior to endotracheal extubation. Ann Surg 1980;191:539–545.

59. Matsushima Y, Jones RL, King EG, Moysa G, Alton JDM. Alterations in pulmonary mechanics and gas exchange during routine fiberoptic bronchoscopy. Chest 1984;86:184–188.

60. England SJ, Bartlett D. Influence of human vocal cord movements on airflow resistance during eupnea. J Appl Physiol 1982;52:773–779.

61. England SJ, Bartlett D. Changes in respiratory movements of the human vocal cords during hyperpnea. J Appl Physiol 1982;52:780–785.

62. Gal TJ, Suratt PM. Resistance to breathing in healthy subjects after endotracheal intubation under topical anesthesia. Anesth Analg 1980;59:270–274.

63. Ferris BG, Mead J, Opie LH. Partitioning of respiratory flow resistance in man. J Appl Physiol 1964;19:653–658.

64. Ross BB, Bramiak R, Rahn H. Physical dynamics of the cough mechanism. J Appl Physiol 1955;8:264–268.

65. Gal TJ. Effects of endotracheal intubation on normal cough performance. Anesthesiology 1980;52:324–329.

66. Leitch AG, Clancy LJ, Costello JF, Flenly DC. Effect of intravenous infusion of salbutamol on ventilatory response to carbon dioxide and hypoxia and on plasma potassium and heart rate in normal man. Br Med J 1976;1:365–367.

67. Gal TJ, Surratt PM, Lu Y. Glycopyrrolate and atropine inhalation: comparative effects on normal airways function. Am Rev Respir Dis 1984;129:871–873.

68. Gal TJ, Surratt PM. Atropine and glycopyrrolate effects on lung mechanics in normal man. Anesth Analg 1980;60:85–90.

69. Keal EE. Physiological and pharmacological control of airway secretions. In: Proctor DF, Reid LM, eds. Respiratory defense mechanism. New York: Marcel Dekker, 1977:357–401.

70. Bukowsky JM, Nakatsu K, Munt PW. Theophylline reassessed. Ann Intern Med 1984;101:63–73.

71. Mackay AD, Baldwin CJ, Tattersfield AE. Action of intravenously administered aminophylline on normal airways. Am Rev Respir Dis 1983;127:609–613.

72. Tobias JD, Kibos KL, Hirshman C. Aminophylline does not inhibit bronchoconstriction during halothame. Anesthesiology 1989;71:723–729.

73. Gong H, Simmons MS, Taashkin DP. Bronchodilator effects of caffeine in coffee. Chest 1986;89:335–342.

74. Littenberg B. Aminophylline treatment in severe acute asthma. A meta analysis. JAMA 1988;259:1678–1684.

75. Dwyer J, Lazarus L, Hickie JB. A study of cortical metabolism in patients with chronic asthma. Aust Ann Med 1967;16:297–303.

76. Morris HG. Mechanism of action and therapeutic role of corticosteroids in asthma. J Allergy Clin Immunol 1985;75:1–13.

77. Schnider SM, Papper EM. Anesthesia for the asthmatic patient. Anesthesiology 1961;22:886–892.

78. Kingston HGG, Hirschman CA. Perioperative management of the patient with asthma. Anesth Analg 1984;63:844–855.

79. Lundy PM, Gowdey CW, Calhoun EH. Tracheal smooth muscle relaxant effect of ketamine. Br J Anaesth 1974;46:333–336.

80. Hirschman CA, Downes H, Farbood A, Bergman NA. Ketamine block of bronchospasm in experimental canine asthma. Br J Anaesth 1979;51:713–718.

81. Huber FC, Reves JG, Guttierrez J, Corssen G. Ketamine: its effect on airway resistance in man. South Med J 1972;65:1176–1180.

82. Weil JV, McCullough RE, Kline JS, Sudal IE. Diminished ventilatory response to hypoxia and hypercapnia after morphine in normal man. N Engl J Med 1975;292:1103–1106.

83. Eschenbacher WL, Bethel RA, Boushey HA, Sheppard D. Morphine sulfate inhibits bronchoconstriction in subjects with mild asthma whose responses are inhibited by atropine. Am Rev Respir Dis 1984;130:363–367.

84. Rosow CE, Moss J, Philbin DM, Savarese JJ. Histamine release during morphine and fentanyl anesthesia. Anesthesiology 1982;56:93–96.

85. Laitinen LA, Empey DW, Poppius H, Lemen RJ, Gold WM, Nadel JA. Effects of intravenous histamine on static lung compliance and airway resistance in normal man. Am Rev Respir Dis 1976;114:291–295.

86. Klioe A, Aviado D. Mechanism for the reduction in pulmonary resistance induced by halothane. J Pharmacol Exp Ther 1967;158:28–35.

87. Hirshman CA, Edelstein G, Peetz S, Wayne R, Downes H. Mechanism of action of inhalational anesthesia on airways. Anesthesiology 1982;56:107–111.

88. Hirschman CA, Bergman NA. Halothane and enflurane protect against bronchospasm in an asthma dog model. Anesth Analg 1978;57:629–633.

89. Brandus V. Joffe S, Benoit CV, Wolff WI. Bronchial spasm during general anesthesia. Can Anaesth Soc J 1970;17:369–274.

90. Downes H, Gerber N, Hirshhman CA. I.V. lignocaine in reflex and allergic bronchoconstriction. Br J Anaesth 1980;52:873–878.

91. Gerbershagen HU, Bergman NA. The effect of d-tubocurarine on respiratory resistance in anesthetized man. Anesthesiology 1967;28:981–984.

92. Crago RR, Bryan AC, Laws AK, Weinstock AE. Respiratory flow resistance after curare and pancuronium measured by forced oscillation. Can Anaesth Soc J 1972;19:607–613.

93. Holtzman MJ, Sheller JR, Dimeo M, Nadel JA, Boushey HA. Effect of ganglionic blockade on bronchial reactivity in atopic subjects. Am Rev Respir Dis 1980;122:17–25.

94. Shah MV, Hirshman CA. Mode of action of halothane on histamine induced constriction in dogs with reactive airways. Anesthesiology 1986;65:170–174.

95. Gold MI. Anesthesia for the asthmatic patient. Anesth Analg 1970;49:881–888.

96. Cooperman LH, Price H. Pulmonary edema in the operative and postoperative period. Ann Surg 1970;172:883–891.

97. Gold MI, Joseph SI. Bilateral tension pneumothorax following induction of anesthesia in two patients with chronic obstructive airway disease. Anesthesiology 1973;38:93–96.

98. Moser K. Pulmonary embolism. Am Rev Respir Dis 1977;115:829–852.

99. Gold MI, Helrich M. Pulmonary mechanics during general anesthesia: V. Status asthamaticus Anesthesiology 1970;32:442–428.

100. Schwartz SH. Treatment of status asthmaticus with halothane. JAMA 1984;251:2688–2689.

101. Parnass SM, Feld J, Chamberlain WH, Segil LJ. Status asthmaticus treated with isoflurane and enflurane. Anesth Analg 1987;66:193–195.

102. Darioli R, Perret C. Mechanical controlled hypoventilation in status asthmaticus. Am Rev Respir Dis 1984;129:385–387.

103. Otis AB, McKerow CB, Bartlett RA, et al. Mechanical factors in distribution of pulmonary ventilation. J Appl Physiol 1956;8:427–443.

104. Connors AF, McCafree RD, Gray BA. Effect of inspiratory flow rate on gas exchange during mechanical ventilation. Am Rev Respir Dis 1981;124:537–543.

105. Tuxen DV, Lane S. The effects of ventilatory pattern on hyperinflation, airway pressures, and circulation in mechanical ventilation of patients with severe airflow obstruction. Am Rev Respir Dis 1987;136:872–879.
106. Crogan SJ, Bishop MJ. Delivery efficiency of metered dose aerosols given via endotracheal tubes. Anesthesiology 1989;70:1008–1010.
107. Stirt JA, Sullivan SF. Aminophylline. Anesth Analg 1981;60:587–560.

SECTION II

Control of Breathing

Chapter 4

Basic Respiratory Control

RESPIRATORY CONTROL SYSTEM

Ventilation—that is, the volume of gas moving into and out of the lungs—is exquisitely matched to metabolic needs. The system that controls this function and adjusts ventilation to keep blood gas tension and acid-base balance within relatively narrow limits is complex but is accomplished by three basic functional elements. These consist of controllers, effectors, and receptors of input or sensors.

Controllers

Within the central nervous system there are two separate areas that serve to control respiration. The first of these, the cerebral controller, actually performs a secondary role. It influences ventilation by superimposing voluntary or behavioral modifications such as voluntary hyperventilation or breath holding. The actual nature of this interaction with the other controller and the effectors is complex and poorly understood.

The primary respiratory controller is composed of neurons in the medulla and pons. Additional neurons in the spinal cord further function to integrate the output of these brain stem areas. Inputs that arrive in the brain stem controller provide the stimuli for automatic breathing. These inputs are integrated and then transmitted via motor neurons to the effectors, the respiratory muscles. The loss of the automatic drive to ventilation is often termed "Ondine's curse" after the German myth of the water nymph Ondine, who took away the automatic or involuntary functions of her unfaithful husband. This loss of automatic breathing can arise from lesions such as tumors, encephalitis, bulbar polio, or interruption of the ninth or tenth cranial nerve pathways. While awake such patients can voluntarily breathe because of the influence of the cerebral controller. During sleep, however, ventilation must be controlled.

Effectors

The rhythmic discharge from the respiratory controllers drives the effectors to achieve ventilation. The effector system consists primarily of the diaphragm and muscles of the chest wall but also includes the muscles of the upper airway. The tonic activity of the latter group, in particular the genioglossus, serves to enlarge the upper airway during each inspiration as the activity of the other respiratory muscles acts to inflate the lungs.

Sensors

The activity of the controllers and effectors is modified by incoming signals from receptors or sensors. These sensors are basically of two types: mechanical and chemical. A numbers of mechanical receptors are found within the upper airway (pharynx, larynx, trachea). Reflexes emanating from these areas are important in affecting tidal volume and respiratory timing (i.e., duration of inspiration and expiration). Information from receptors in the chest wall is believed to be important in the sensation of dyspnea. Finally, the stretch, irritant, and J receptors mentioned previously with respect to bronchial activity (see Chapter 3) also play a reflex role in breathing.

Since the respiratory controller is primarily concerned with maintaining normal gas exchange and acid-base balance, its principal input is derived from chemical sensors. These include both central and peripheral chemoreceptors. The area of central chemosensitivity appears to lie on the ventrolateral surface of the medulla.[1] Breathing is stimulated largely in response to CO_2, which crosses the blood-brain barrier and changes the hydrogen ion content at these sites. Most evidence indicates that these chemoreceptor structures are separate from the brain stem respiratory neurons that function as the respiratory controllers.[2]

The peripheral chemoreceptors, the carotid and aortic bodies, are small 1- to 2-mm node-like structures closely related to each carotid sinus and to the aortic arch. These tiny structures are extremely vascular and have extremely high rates of blood flow and metabolic oxygen consumption compared to other tissues. Of the two the carotid body appears to be more important. Its neural activity is increased by arterial hypoxemia, hypercapnia, and acidemia. The acute ventilatory response to lack of oxygen requires intact, functioning carotid bodies. The response to CO_2 increase will remain relatively intact after peripheral chemoreceptor denervation such as can result from bilateral carotid endarterectomy.[3] Approximately 80 to 85% of the ventilatory response to CO_2 arises from the central chemoreceptors. Thus, denervation of both carotid bodies results in a 15 to 20% decrease in resting ventilation and a small (5 to 6 mm Hg) rise in resting $Paco_2$.

CHEMICAL REGULATION OF VENTILATION

Although the analysis of the system that controls breathing can be subdivided into chemical and neural elements, clinical appraisal of the neural control system is much more difficult and hazardous. The chemical control system responds to three basic physiological stimuli: increases in the partial pressure of CO_2, increases in hydrogen ion concentration (decreased blood pH), and decreases in arterial Po_2.

Effects of Hypercapnia on Breathing

Metabolically produced carbon dioxide relies on ventilation for its removal. If ventilation is reduced $Paco_2$ will rise. Similarly, if ventilation is voluntarily or reflexly increased $Paco_2$ will decrease. The reciprocal relationship between ventilation and CO_2 is described by a rectangular hyperbola. For CO_2 excretion (Fig. 4.1) it is apparent from the diagram that a doubling of ventilation results in a halving of CO_2 tension, while CO_2 tension doubles if ventilation is halved. An average normal man has an alveolar ventilation of about 4 liters/min and a resting $Paco_2$ near 4 mm Hg as shown in the figure as point *A*.

In the same normal individual, inhalation of CO_2 increases ventilation, which rises in nearly linear fashion with changes in $Paco_2$. Stimulation to breathe depends on the hydrogen ion concentration in the extracellular fluid surrounding the CNS chemoreceptors near the ventrolateral surface of the medulla. The change in hydrogen ion concentration as a result of inhaling CO_2 depends somewhat on the concentration of bicarbonate in the extracelluar fluid. Alterations of bicarbonate levels in blood or cerebrospinal fluid from metabolic disturbances can therefore modify the ventilatory response to CO_2.

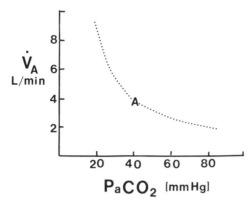

Figure 4.1. CO_2 excretion hyperbola describing the reciprocal relationship between alveolar ventilation ($\dot{V}A$) and arterial CO_2 tension ($Paco_2$). The curve assumes a constant CO_2 production. Under normal resting conditions the relationship lies at point *A*. (Reproduced with permission from Gal TJ. Respiratory physiology during anesthesia. In: Kaplan JA, ed. Thoracic anesthesia. 2nd ed. New York: Churchill Livingstone, 1990, Chapter 8.)

The central chemoreceptors account for about 80% of the total increase in ventilation during inhalation of CO_2. The remaining 20% increase seems to arise from stimulation of peripheral chemoreceptors.

Effects of Hypoxia on Breathing

The ventilatory response to decreases in inspired oxygen tension tends to be hyperbolic (Fig. 4.2) such that decreases in oxygen tension exert a greater effect on ventilation when hypoxemia is severe as opposed to mild reductions in oxygen supply. The curvilinear relationship can be conveniently converted to a straight line by plotting ventilation against the reciprocal of arterial oxygen tension ($1/Pao_2$) or, as is more common, against arterial O_2 saturation. The nice linear relationship with O_2 saturation suggests that ventilation may be influenced primarily by the oxygen content. Most studies, however, point to arterial oxygen tension as the stimulus to the peripheral chemoreceptors. This is underscored by the effect of inhaling carbon monoxide, which markedly affects O_2 content. The latter has little or no effect on ventilation, since Pao_2 is not affected.[4]

The hypoxic ventilatory response is mediated by the peripheral chemoreceptors in the carotid body. In their absence the hypoxic ventilatory drive is lost and hypoxia may exert a depressant action on the central chemoreceptors. The carotid bodies exert only a subtle influence on resting ventilation when Pao_2 is greater than 60 mm Hg. Below this level ventilation increases dramatically in hyperbolic fashion, whereas at a Pao_2 of 200 mm Hg or more the carotid body discharge diminishes to a minimal level.

An important interaction occurs between the two major ventilatory stimulants of hypoxia and hypercapnia. The presence of hypoxia enhances the ventilatory response to CO_2. Similarly, an increase in CO_2 results in a greater sen-

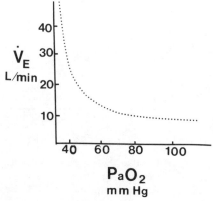

Figure 4.2. Effects of decreasing arterial oxygen tension (Pao_2) on minute ventilation ($\dot{V}E$). The hyperbolic plot can be lineralized by plotting $\dot{V}E$ against the reciprocal of Pao_2 or against O_2 saturation. (Reproduced with permission from Gal TJ. Respiratory physiology during anesthesia. In: Kaplan JA, ed. Thoracic anesthesia. 2nd ed. New York: Churchill Livingstone, 1990, Chapter 8.)

sitivity to hypoxia. These interactive effects require an intact central as well as peripheral chemoreceptor function.

Effects of Metabolic Acidosis

A decrease in arterial pH from metabolic acidosis with normal Pao_2 and $Paco_2$ stimulates ventilation primarily by the effect of the acidemia on the peripheral chemoreceptors (carotid bodies). This arises from the concept that neither hydrogen nor bicarbonate ions readily cross the blood-brain barrier and is supported by observations in dogs that carotid body denervation attenuates and delays the response.[5] Biscoe et al.[6] demonstrated in cats that a change of 0.20 pH units (7.45 to 7.25) increased carotid body neural output 2 to 3 times. This doubling of ventilation is roughly equivalent to that seen when Pao_2 decreases from normal to about 40 or 50 mm Hg.

Knill and Clement[7] noted approximately a doubling of ventilation in normoxic, normocarbic volunteers as the hydrogen ion concentration was increased about 13 nmol/liter (about 0.12 units pH decrease). This response was attenuated by hyperoxia and enhanced by hypoxia, again attesting to the interaction of these stimuli at the peripheral chemoreceptor.

All in all, for the same degree of acidemia or pH change, the addition of CO_2 evokes a larger increment in ventilation than does the addition of fixed acid. The initial response to acute metabolic acidosis is weak because as $Paco_2$ decreases from carotid body stimulation, CO_2 tension in the cerebrospinal fluid decreases and pH increases. Thus, the strong peripheral stimulation of the hydrogen ion is offset by a central alkalosis and reduced stimulus to the medullary chemoreceptors. Gradually after several hours, bicarbonate levels decrease and permit cerebrospinal fluid pH to decrease back toward its normal value. As a result, central chemoreceptor activity is restored to normal.

Effect of Metabolic Alkalosis

Unlike the relatively consistent compensatory mechanism in metabolic acidosis, those associated with metabolic alkalosis are rather inconsistent and controversial. The observations indicate that metabolic alkalosis is not a well-defined, limited entity and the differences relate to the manner in which the alkalosis is produced. Respiratory compensation (i.e., hypoventilation) is minimal or absent when alkalosis is associated with hypokalemia, as with diuretics. Compensation was greatest when alkalosis was induced by agents that increased buffer base in all body fluid compartments.[8]

MEASUREMENT OF VENTILATORY RESPONSES

Ventilatory control mechanisms can be assessed at rest but are usually characterized by the response to standard perturbations or stimuli. These usually consist of induced changes in arterial CO_2 or O_2 tension. The output of the respiratory neurons or the ventilatory drive is usually reflected by increases in minute ventilation in normals. However factors that increase the mechanical work of breathing may modify the ventilation that results from a given amount of respiratory stimulation in certain disease states. Thus it is important to assess respiratory muscle strength and evaluate other aspects of respiratory mechanics by spirometry in such patients prior to interpreting ventilatory responsiveness.

Sensitivity to Carbon Dioxide

As alveolar or arterial CO_2 tension increases, the increased ventilation resulting from this acute hypercapnia is linearly related to the CO_2 stimulus. Because hypoxia affects CO_2 sensitivity, the response is usually measured with oxygen-enriched mixtures so that arterial oxygen tension is greater than 150 mm Hg. Thus the central medullary chemoreceptor activity is responsible for the increase in ventilation.

Various techniques have been used to test the chemosensitivity to carbon dioxide. The techniques, which include both steady-state and rebreathing methods, differ solely in the manner in which hypercapnia is produced.

Steady-State Technique.   This method relies on measuring the ventilatory response to a steadily maintained CO_2 stimulus. Thus ventilation and CO_2 levels are measured for 10 to 15 minutes after a gas mixture containing increased CO_2 is breathed. Usually three such gas mixtures (3, 5, and 7% CO_2) are used. Each is breathed for the prolonged period to ensure that $Paco_2$ and hydrogen ion concentration have equilibrated and are similar in the environment of the medullary chemoreceptors. Such equilibration may be difficult to achieve in patients with pulmonary disease. Because of the prolonged equilibration required with the steady-state technique, a response curve generated at two levels of CO_2 stimulation (dual isohypercapnia) has been used.[9]

Rebreathing.   Because of its time-consuming nature, the steady-state method has experienced limited use clinically. Currently, the most widely used clinical technique of CO_2 response testing is the rebreathing method originally described by Read.[10] He demonstrated that the response can be determined rapidly as subjects rebreathe from a small bag or spirometer containing 7% CO_2 and 93% O_2. The rate at which alveolar and arterial CO_2 tensions rise is largely a function of the volume contained in the rebreathing bag. Usually this is equivalent to the subject's vital capacity plus 1 liter (6 to 7 liters). The 7% CO_2 approximates mixed venous levels and expedites the equilibration of CO_2 among alveolar (end-tidal), arterial, and brain compartments. This initial equilibration is further enhanced by having subjects take two or three vital-capacity breaths with the CO_2 mixture prior to rebreathing. Since CO_2 is not eliminated from the system during rebreathing, arterial and alveolar CO_2 are not affected by the level or pattern of ventilation. Rather, they rise about 3 to 6 mm Hg per minute and provide an open physiologic control loop to stimulate ventilation.

This open loop is advantageous because, unlike in the steady-state method, changes in ventilation do not affect end-tidal or alveolar CO_2 tensions.[11] Furthermore, ventilation can be measured over a rather large range of CO_2 tension in a brief period (5 to 6 minutes).

Sensitivity to Hypoxia

Steady-State Techniques. Much like the responses to CO_2, the ventilatory responses to hypoxia have been evaluated by steady-state and non–steady-state techniques. In the steady-state techniques gas mixtures containing various O_2 concentrations are breathed while CO_2 is added to the inspired gas as ventilation increases to hold alveolar CO_2 constant.[12] Ventilation can then be plotted as a function of oxygen tension at that particular CO_2 concentration. An alternative approach determines the influence of hypoxia on steady-state CO_2 responses. Here the hypercapneic inspired mixtures are breathed at high (Po_2 = 200 mm Hg) and low (Po_2 = 40 mm Hg) oxygen concentrations. The major difficulty with such steady-state techniques is the prolonged hypoxia that is required. Thus their use is largely confined to the experimental laboratory area, and their clinical utility is limited at best.

Non–Steady-State Technique. Such tests involve rapid change in oxygen in the inspired gas mixture. This takes advantage of the quick equilibration of peripheral chemoreceptors with inspired oxygen tension. The rapid changes in oxygen tension require a rapidly responding O_2 analyzer or an accurate, responsive ear oximeter. Progressive hypoxia may be produced by rebreathing a mixture of air and CO_2. Isocapneic conditions are maintained by a soda lime CO_2 absorber.[13] Another method uses progressive addition of nitrogen to the breathing mixture to stimulate respiration.[14] The latter procedure is performed over a 20-minute period. To avoid any possible direct depressant effects of hypoxia on the central chemoreceptors, Edelman et al.[15] attempted to achieve a briefer exposure. They used several (usually one to five) breaths of nitrogen with no attempt to control CO_2. In a matter of seconds O_2 saturation decreased and ventilation increased. Hypoxic sensitivity was expressed as the maximal ventilation produced in response to the minimal O_2 saturation after several exposures to inspired N_2 breaths.

Sensitivity to Metabolic Acidosis

The ventilatory response to metabolic acidemia, which is a function of peripheral carotid body stimulation, has received far less attention than the responses to hypoxia and hypercapnia. Such acidosis has been produced by infusion of ammonium chloride and more recently by L-arginine hydrochloride.[7] The most important factor to remember with stimulation from metabolic acidosis is the significant interaction of hypoxemia and hypercapnia at the peripheral chemoreceptor. Thus hypercapnia and hypoxia augment the response, while hypocapnia and hyperoxia attenuate the stimulus to ventilation.

Ventilatory Indices of Chemosensitivity

Carbon Dioxide Response.   The two basic variables of ventilatory control (i.e., resting ventilation and $Paco_2$) may be highly variable and only slightly affected when the ventilatory control system is significantly altered.[16] Nevertheless, they have been advocated as indices of ventilatory control[17] largely because the CO_2 stimulus in most CO_2 response studies is not the same as the more relevant metabolic CO_2 stimulus.[18]

Conventional means of expressing CO_2 sensitivity use a plot of the CO_2 load or stimulus on the abscissa and ventilation on the ordinate. The latter values are obtained from actual data points with steady-state techniques, while least squares linear regression determines the plot with rebreathing data. The carbon dioxide stimulus on the abscissa has included inspired CO_2 concentration, end-tidal tension, or arterial tension. Most frequently end-tidal tension is used; however, arterial tension ($Paco_2$) may be the most accurate reflection of the CO_2 stimulus, particularly if pulmonary disease is present. The ordinate on the carbon dioxide ventilation plot is provided by respiratory minute volume ($\dot{V}E$). The hyperoxic carbon dioxide sensitivity is expressed as the increment in $\dot{V}E$ (in liters per minute) per increment in $Paco_2$ (in millimeters of mercury). This can be quantitated by the equation:

$$\dot{V}E = S(Paco_2 - B)$$

where S is the slope of the relationship between $\dot{V}E$ and $Paco_2$ and B is the intercept on the x axis. The steeper the slope, the more vigorous the response to CO_2 (*A* in Fig. 4.3). As such it provides a measure of the gain of the control system.

In most normal young adults the slope of the CO_2 response ranges from 1.5 to 5.0 liters/min/mm Hg CO_2.[19] Many of the interindividual differences in the response relate to the tidal volume response during rebreathing. In general, the lowest ventilatory responses occurred in those whose tidal volumes were the smallest.[20]

Changes in CO_2 sensitivity can be indicated by slope changes in the response. However, some factors, such as pharmacological intervention, may alter CO_2 sensitivity without changing the slope. In this case the shift of the CO_2 response can be characterized by a term referred to as displacement (*B* in Fig. 4.3). This is the shift across the x axis in mm Hg CO_2 at a constant ordinate ($\dot{V}E$) value, usually 20 or 30 liters/min. Another expression for the shift of the CO_2 response curve uses a change in ordinate ($\dot{V}E$) at a constant CO_2 value (*C* in Fig. 4.3). Often 60 mm Hg is used and the term referred to as the $\dot{V}E_{60}$. Another interesting term represents an extrapolation of the CO_2 response curve to zero ventilation on the CO_2 axis (*D* in Fig. 4.3). This "apneic threshold" represents the CO_2 level at which apnea should occur from hyperventilation. This value is not easily obtainable in awake persons and may not provide any more information than the resting. $Paco_2$.

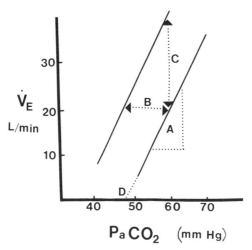

Figure 4.3. Hypercapneic ventilatory response expressed as increase in minute ventilation ($\dot{V}E$) as a function of increased arterial CO_2 tension (Pa_{CO_2}). *A*, slope of the response; *B*, displacement of the response (i.e., a change in the abscissa at a constant ordinate value); *C*, change in ordinate at a constant abscissal value; *D*, apneic threshold. (Reproduced with permission from Gal TJ. Respiratory physiology during anesthesia. In: Kaplan JA, ed. Thoracic anesthesia. 2nd ed. New York: Churchill Livingstone, 1990, Chapter 8.)

Hypoxic Response.   Ideally, the hypoxic ventilatory response should be expressed as a change in ventilation for a change in the stimulus (decreased O_2). However, the curvilinear nature of the relationship renders it complex and not easily characterized by a single index. One early index compared the ratio of the slopes of two CO_2 response curves, one performed in the presence of hypoxia (Pa_{O_2} = 40 mm Hg) and the other normoxia (Pa_{O_2} = 150 mm Hg).[21] This dimensionless ratio has little physiological meaning and is highly dependent on the hypercapneic response.

Severinghaus[22] introduced an index termed $\Delta\dot{V}_{40}$, which was expressed in liters per minute. This represented the increase in minute ventilation that occurred as oxygen tension was reduced from above 200 mm Hg to 40 mm Hg with normocapnia. At an oxygen tension of 40 mm Hg the ventilatory response is rather steep (Fig. 4.4). Thus the potential for error exists in estimating the actual ventilation value, since small decreases in Po_2 are associated with rather large increases in ventilation. The $\Delta\dot{V}_{40}$ can also be estimated from the two CO_2 response curves, one performed with normoxia and the other at hypoxic level (Pa_{O_2} = 40 mm Hg). Ventilations measured at an isocapneic point (Pa_{CO_2} = 40 mm Hg) can thus be compared.

The ventilatory response to hypoxia can be linearized by plotting ventilation against the reciprocal of Po_2 or, more conveniently, by relating the change in ventilation to arterial oxyhemoglobin saturation (Fig. 4.4). Thus the hypoxic response can be quantitated as $\Delta\dot{V}$/% desaturation. Although the latter index is the simplest means of quantitating the hypoxic response, a more complex description of the hyperbolic relationship between ventilation ($\dot{V}E$) and oxygen

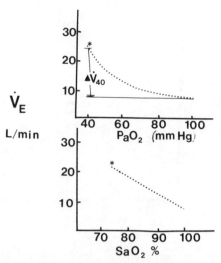

Figure 4.4. The hyperbolic response to hypoxia can be quantitated as $\Delta\dot{V}_{40}$, the increase in ventilation ($\dot{V}_E$) at a hypoxic level ($Pao_2 = 40$ mm Hg) compared to normoxia. Note that the increased $\dot{V}_E$ is linearly related to arterial O_2 saturation ($Sao_2\%$). At a Pao_2 of 40 mm Hg the blood is roughly 25% desaturated ($Sao_2 = 75\%$). Thus ventilation at this point and at Pao_2 of 40 mm Hg are nearly identical (*). (Reproduced with permission from Gal TJ. Respiratory physiology during anesthesia. In: Kaplan JA, ed. Thoracic anesthesia. 2nd ed. New York: Churchill Livingstone, 1990, Chapter 8.)

tension (Pao_2) is equally popular. Parameter A is used to characterize the shape of the curve that is expressed mathematically by the equation:

$$\dot{V}_E = \dot{V}_O + A/(Pao_2 - 32)$$

$\dot{V}_O$ is the asymptote for ventilation; 32 is the asymptote for Pao_2 at which ventilation is assumed to be infinite. The magnitude of A is related to the briskness of the response.

In normal subjects the ventilatory response to hypoxia appears to be more variable than the hypercapneic response. For example, while the mean value for parameter A was 186, the range of values was from 69 to 410.[23] In terms of desaturation, hypoxic sensitivity ranged from 0.16 to 1.35 liters/min per 1% desaturation (mean = 0.6),[24] while $\Delta\dot{V}_{40}$ values ranged from 5.4 to 64.8 liters/min.[25] Certain mathematical interrelationships can be constructed for these three indices. For example, since normal blood undergoes a 25% desaturation at a Pao_2 of 40 mm Hg, the $\Delta\dot{V}/1\%$ desaturation and $\Delta\dot{V}_{40}$ are related by a factor of 25 to 1 such that $\Delta\dot{V}_{40}/25 = \Delta\dot{V}/1\%$ desaturation. Also, if $Pao_2 = 40$ mm Hg is substituted into the equation containing parameter A, the following relationship results: $A = \Delta\dot{V}_{40} \times 8$.

Other Indices of Respiratory Center Output

Ventilatory Drive and Timing. Traditional methods for measuring ventilatory drive have used the measurement of minute ventilation to express the effects of stimuli on respiratory center output. In most patients with normal respiratory system mechanics such measurement of the ventilatory response provides a reasonably valid reflection of respiratory drive. Further valuable analysis can be obtained by analyzing the pattern and timing of the response. Indeed, the pattern, which consists of tidal volume (V_T), can result from changes in the duration of inspiration (T_I) or by change in mean inspiratory flow (V_T/T_I). The total duration of each respiratory cycle (T_{TOT}) is a combination of the duration of inspiration (T_I) as well as expiration (T_E). Since respiratory frequency (f) is essentially equal to $60/T_{TOT}$, respiratory frequency can be altered by changes in T_I, T_E, or both. Each breathing cycle has been characterized as the result of two basic mechanisms, drive and timing.[26] The V_T/T_I reflects the activity of the driving mechanism, whereas T_I/T_{TOT}, the fraction of the total respiratory cycle occupied by inspiration, is an index of timing.

Occlusion Pressure ($P_{0.1}$). The negative pressure generated at the mouth during the first 100 milliseconds of inspiration against an occluded airway ($P_{0.1}$) has gained widespread acceptance as a clinical correlate of central respiratory drive. The $P_{0.1}$ reflects respiratory drive in normal subjects and those with mechanical dysfunction of the respiratory system. Although the measurement has some limitations as a direct index of inspiratory neural drive,[27] it is useful to identify whether ventilatory failure is the result of abnormal respiratory mechanics or an abnormality of respiratory control.

Diaphragmatic Electromyogram. The generation of inspiratory pressure such as the $P_{0.1}$ requires intact innervation of the diaphragm. Thus, diaphragmatic electromyography would appear to be a valid indicator of central chemosensitivity. However, reproducible recordings are difficult to obtain with esophageal electrodes because changes in position can often vary the magnitude of response more than ventilatory stimuli. The discomfort associated with the electrodes has also hampered their widespread use. Fortunately, changes in $P_{0.1}$ correlate favorably with this invasive technique.[28]

REFERENCES

1. Mitchell RA, Loeschke HH, Massion WH et al. Respiratory response mediated through superficial chemosensitive areas of the medulla. J Appl Physiol 1963;18:523–533.
2. Mitchell RA, Herbert DA. The effect of carbon dioxide on the membrane potential of medullary respiratory neurons. Brain Res 1974;75:345–349.
3. Wade JG, Larson CP, Hickey RF, Ehrenfeld WK, Severinghaus JW. Effect of carotid endarterectomy on carotid chemoreceptor and baroreceptor function in man. N Engl J Med 1970;282:823–829.
4. Dejours P. Chemoreflexes in breathing. Physiol Rev 1962;42:335–358.
5. Mitchell RA. The regulation of respiration in metabolic acidosis and alkalosis. In: Brooks CMC, Kao FF, Lloyd BB, eds. Cerebrospinal fluid and the regulation of ventilation. Oxford, England: Blackwell, 1965: 109–131.
6. Biscoe TJ, Purves MJ, Sampson SR. The frequency of nerve impulses in single carotid body chemoreceptor afferent fibers recorded in vivo with intact circulation. J Physiol (Lond) 1970;208:121–131.
7. Knill RL, Clement JL. Ventilatory responses to acute metabolic acidemia in humans awake, sedated, and anesthetized with halothane. Anesthesiology 1985;62:745–753.

8. Goldring RM, Cannon PJ, Heineman HO, Fishman AP. Respiratory adjustment to chronic metabolic alkalosis in man. J Clin Invest 1968;47:188–202.

9. Gross JB, Zebrowski ME, Carel WD, Gardner S, Smith TC. Time course of ventilatory depression after thiopental and midazolam in normal subjects and in patients with chronic obstructive pulmonary disease. Anesthesiology 1983;58:540–544.

10. Read DJC. A clinical method for assessing the ventilatory response to carbon dioxide. Australas Ann Med 1967;16:20–32.

11. Rebuck AS, Read J. Patterns of ventilatory response to carbon dioxide during recovery from severe asthma. Clin Sci 1971;41:13–21.

12. Lloyd BB, Cunningham DJC. A quantitative approach to the regulation of human respiration. In: Cunningham DJC, Lloyd BB, eds. The regulation of human respiration. Oxford, England: Blackwell, 1963: 331–349.

13. Rebuck AS, Campbell EJM. A clinical method for assessing the ventilatory response to hypoxia. Am Rev Respir Dis 1974;109:345–350.

14. Weil JV, Byrne-Quinn E, Sodal I, et al. Hypoxic ventilatory drive in normal man. J Clin Invest 1970;49:1061–1072.

15. Edelman NH, Epstein PE, Lahiri S, Cherniack NS. The ventilatory responses to transient hypoxia and hypercapnia in man. Respir Physiol 1973;17:302–314.

16. Gross JB. Resting ventilation measurements may be misleading. Anesthesiology 1984;61:110.

17. Knill RL. Wresting or resting ventilation. Anesthesiology 1983;59:559–600.

18. Stremel RW, Huntsman DJ, Casaburi R, Whipp BJ, Wasserman K. Control of ventilation during intravenous CO_2 loading in the awake dog. J Appl Physiol 1978;44:311–316.

19. Irsigler GB. Carbon dioxide response lines in young adults: the limits of the normal response. Am Rev Respir Dis 1976;114:529–536.

20. Rebuck AS, Rigg JRA, Kangalee M, Pengelly LD. Control of tidal volume during rebreathing. J Appl Physiol 1973;37:475–478.

21. Nielson M, Smith H. Studies on the regulation of respiration in acute hypoxia. Acta Physiol Scand 1952;24:293–313.

22. Severinghaus J, Bainton CR, Carcelena A. Respiratory insensitivity to hypoxia in chronically hypoxic man. Respir Physiol 1966;1:308–334.

23. Hirschman CA, McCullough RE, Weil JV. Normal values for hypoxic and hypercapneic ventilatory drives in man. J Appl Physiol 1975;38:1095–1098.

24. Rebuck AS, Woodley WE. Ventilatory effects of hypoxia and their dependence on P_{CO_2}. J Appl Physiol 1975;38:16–19.

25. Kronenberg RS, Hamilton FN, Gabel R, Hickey R, Read DJC, Severinghaus J. Comparison of three methods for quantitating respiratory response to hypoxia. Respir Physiol 1972;16:109–125.

26. Milic-Emili J, Grunstein MM. Drive and timing components of ventilation. Chest 1976;70 (suppl):131–133.

27. Milic-Emili J. Recent advances in clinical assessment of control of breathing. Lung 1982;160:1–17.

28. Lopata M, Evanich MJ, Lourenco RV. Relationship between mouth occlusion pressure and electrical activity of the diaphragm: effects of flow restive loading. Am Rev Respir Dis 1977;116:449–455.

Chapter 5

Control of Breathing in Normal and Disease States

CONTROL OF BREATHING IN NORMAL STATES

Normal Variations with Age

Alterations in the ventilatory responses to hypoxia and hypercapnia have been demonstrated in many disease states. However, even in the normal population the wide variations may be attributed to a host of factors that modify the responses. For example, advancing age is associated with a gradual decline in pulmonary function manifested by decreasing vital capacity, maximal flow rates, and arterial oxygen tension. In a study of normal elderly persons (ages 65 to 79) the ventilatory responses to both hypoxia and hypercapnia were reduced to about half those seen in normal younger counterparts.[1, 2] Since occlusion pressure responses were reduced to the same extent as the ventilatory responses,[1] the differences could not be attributed to mechanical factors but rather were the result of altered chemosensitivity.

At the other extreme of age, the normal newborn sustains its higher oxygen demands per unit mass through an increased $\dot{V}E$, decreased resting P_{CO_2}, and a shift in the CO_2 response curve to the left.[3] The slope of the CO_2 response is similar to that for adults but appears to be a function of gestational age. For example, slopes for term infants were 5 times those for preterm (29 to 32 weeks) infants.[4] In the latter group, hypoxia depressed rather than augmented the CO_2 response.[5] The response to hypoxia in normal newborns is not sustained but rather is biphasic, i.e., it increases initially but then decreases to an intermediate level slightly above baseline. The hypoxic response in adults is also biphasic, but the time course is different.[6] In infants ventilation begins to decrease after 2 to 5 minutes of isocapneic hypoxia, whereas in adults the high level of ventilation is sustained for 20 to 25 minutes before decreasing.

85

Hereditary Aspects of Ventilatory Responses

Numerous observations have suggested that there is a familial influence on the determination of ventilatory drive. Low ventilatory responses to CO_2 and a diminished response to added airway resistance were characteristic of parents whose children succumbed to the sudden infant death syndrome.[7] Normal adult offspring of patients with hypercapnia due to chronic obstructive airway disease had decreased responses to hypoxia and hypercapnia when compared to offspring of patients with similar obstruction but normocapnia.[8] For the most part, heredity appears to influence the hypoxic response more consistently than the hypercapneic response. This is evident in the case of identical twins[4] and endurance athletes.[9] In the latter group of long-distance runners, familial factors appear to play a major role in their decreased hypoxic ventilatory response.

Acclimatization to Altitude

While the reduced hypoxic response appears to benefit the endurance athlete at sea level, at high altitude the relative hypoventilation is detrimental and is more likely to be associated with acute mountain sickness.[10] Because of the low ambient O_2 tension at extreme altitude, a brisk ventilatory response is required for adequate arterial oxygenation. Schoene[11] has demonstrated that subjects who ascend to altitude best have brisk responses to hypoxia in contrast to those of distance runners (Fig. 5.1). The response to hypercapnia in these same climbing subjects also tended to be significantly higher than that of the runners. Subsequently Schoene demonstrated that exercise performance on Mount Everest correlated with the briskness of the ventilatory response to hypoxia.[12]

Longstanding exposure to high altitude or to low arterial O_2 tension, as in the case of cyanotic heart disease, appears to be associated with decreased ventilatory sensitivity to hypoxia. The reduced sensitivity is not present in children native to high altitude but rather appears to be acquired over many years.[13] Once established, this densensitization was thought to be irreversible. This appears to be the case with altitude dwellers, but in some patients with cyanotic heart disease, surgical correction of the cardiac defects improved the hypoxic response.[14]

Sleep and the Normal Ventilatory Response

Much of the evidence in normal adult humans indicates that compared to wakefulness, there is a slight decrease in the slope of the ventilatory response to CO_2 in quiet or non–rapid eye movement (NREM) sleep.[15] Because resting ventilation is decreased there must be a shift in the position of the response curve to a higher CO_2 level as well. The hypoxic response measured as $\Delta \dot{V}/\%$ desaturation also decreased to two-thirds of its awake value during NREM

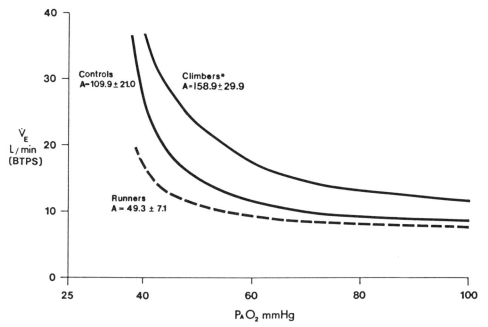

Figure 5.1. Hypoxic ventilatory responses contrasting the brisk response of climbers with the rather blunted response of runners. The hyperbolic relationship of ventilation ($\dot{V}_E$) and arterial oxygen tension (Pao_2) is indicated by parameter A. (From Schoene RB., Control of ventilation in climbers to extreme altitude. J Appl Physiol 1982;53:886–890.)

sleep and was depressed significantly further during REM sleep.[16] This can account for some of the sleep-related hypoxemia seen in some disease states and in normals. Particularly noteworthy are preterm infants, who spend 50 to 60% of their time in REM sleep, during which they are prone to alveolar hypoventilation and apneic spells.

Exercise and Metabolic Influences on Ventilatory Responses

The ventilatory response to exercise is complex, since subjects progress through several phases from rest to maximum exercise. During moderate exercise, normocapnia is accompanied by an increased ventilation, which is directly related to CO_2 production. Only with heavy exercise does a disproportional hyperventilation occur. This presumably results from a metabolic acidosis that stimulates carotid body peripheral chemoreceptors, since hyperpnea with maximum exercise is reduced in subjects after carotid body resection.[17] For the most part, the ventilatory response to exercise tends to reflect the underlying responses to hypoxia and hypercapnia. In many athletes, for example, these ventilatory responses and the response to exercise are blunted to a similar degree.[18]

There are numerous metabolic and humoral factors that alter ventilatory responsiveness. Among these is progesterone, which is implicated as the cause of hyperventilation during pregnancy[19] and during the menstrual cycle.[20] Indeed, in healthy women Schoene et al.[21] have shown that both ventilatory drive and exercise ventilation increase during the luteal phase when compared to the follicular phase.

Other factors, such as increased body temperature, increase the ventilatory response to hypoxia and hypercapnia in humans.[22] Whether this is a direct effect of temperature or an indirect one as a result of metabolism is unknown. Indeed, hypermetabolism, whether induced by feeding[23] or by intravenous infusion,[24] is associated with increased resting ventilation and increased sensitivity to CO_2 and hypoxia.

CONTROL OF BREATHING IN DISEASE STATES

Chronic Obstructive Pulmonary Disease

Hypercapnia and hypoxemia often develop in patients with chronic obstructive pulmonary disease (COPD) as their disease advances. These gas exchange abnormalities have been attributed to mechanical limitations,[25] poor matching of ventilation and perfusion,[26] as well as decreased sensitivity to hypoxia and hypercapnia as ventilatory stimuli. Patients with COPD frequently have blunted ventilatory responses. Interpretation of these responses requires indices other than minute ventilation because of the mechanical limitations imposed by disease. Other indices of respiratory center activity, such as phrenic electromyography[27] and occlusion pressure $(P_{0.1})$,[28] have been used to distinguish the patients who cannot breathe from those who will not breathe. In addition, the chemical and neurogenic depression can be more precisely identified if the ventilatory responses in patients with airflow obstruction are corrected for variations in maximum voluntary ventilation.[29]

In patients with airway obstruction hypercapneic ventilatory responses tend to be decreased compared to normals. In normocapneic patients the CO_2 responses in terms of electromyographic activity[29] and occlusion pressures[30] appear to be essentially normal. The occlusion pressures $(P_{0.1})$ during quiet room air breathing and at elevated CO_2 levels are increased and suggest heightened respiratory center activity (*B* in Fig. 5.2). By comparison, patients with resting hypercapnia demonstrate a reduced slope of the occlusion pressure response (*C* in Fig. 5.2) as well as the ventilatory response. Note that, although the $P_{0.1}$ at rest is higher than in normals (*A* in Fig. 5.2), the values with further increases in CO_2 are markedly depressed compared to normals.

Numerous observations in COPD patients have demonstrated that patients with hypercapnia tend to have a shorter duration of inspiration, smaller tidal volumes, and more rapid respiratory rates than their normocapneic counterparts.[31] This pattern of breathing tends to increase the dead space to tidal volume ratio. Thus, despite increases in minute ventilation, alveolar ventilation decreases and CO_2 retention is more likely to develop. For the most

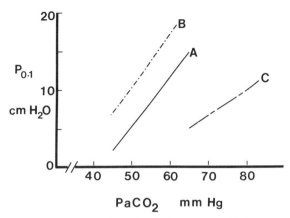

Figure 5.2. Diagrammatic representation of occlusion pressure ($P_{0.1}$) responses to CO_2 in normals (A), patients with chronic obstructive pulmonary disease (COPD) with normocapnia (B), and COPD patients with resting hypercapnia (C).

part this CO_2 retention is associated with more hypoxemia than that seen in normocapneic patients. The hypoxemia may in fact be responsible for the characteristic pattern of rapid, shallow breathing.[32]

In patients who are chronically hypoxemic the normal augmentation of the hypercapneic ventilatory response by hypoxia is significantly attentuated.[33] This reduced ventilatory response correlates with the degree of airway obstruction and suggests that mechanical limitations are important. However, other investigators have shown that hypoxemic patients have reduced responses to hypoxia, in terms of both ventilatory and occlusion pressure ($P_{0.1}$) responses.[34] Ventilatory responses to CO_2 are depressed in the same patients, but $P_{0.1}$ responses are not.

The decreased hypoxic response in hypoxemic patients might be likened to that which develops in high-altitude dwellers or is seen in cyanotic patients with congenital heart defects. On the other hand, one could postulate that the decreased hypoxic response preceded the onset of lung disease and contributed to the hypoxemia.

The finding of depressed responses to hypoxia in hypoxemic patients compared to patients without hypoxemia but with similar degrees of chronic airway obstruction[35] raises serious questions about the mechanism of CO_2 narcosis as a result of correcting hypoxemia. The deleterious effects of administering oxygen-enriched mixtures to hypoxemic, hypercapneic patients has been attributed to removal of the hypoxic ventilatory drive. One would therefore suspect that such patients have a blunted CO_2 response but an intact hypoxic response.

The administration of an oxygen-enriched mixture ($F_{IO_2} = 0.4$) to 20 patients with COPD in early stages of acute respiratory failure ($Pa_{O_2} < 40$ mm Hg; $Pa_{CO_2} > 60$ mm Hg) resulted in a slight (14%) decrease in minute ventilation ($\dot{V}_E$) and a 12% increase in Pa_{CO_2}.[35] Although these average changes appear to be proportional, there was no relationship in individual patients between changes in $\dot{V}E$ and concomitant changes in $Paco_2$. These findings, as well as the effects of 100% O_2 in another group of similar patients[36] and observations in stable COPD patients,[37] suggest that hypercapnia induced by hyperoxia is not primarily related to altered respiratory drive but rather is the result of further impairment in gas exchange. The increase in alveolar O_2 tension reduced the hypoxic pulmonary vasoconstriction that normally maintains ventilation-perfusion matching. This shift of blood to poorly ventilated areas results in an increased dead space (VD). The increase in VD could also be partially related to the Haldane effect, which results in displacement of CO_2 from oxygenated blood and thus increases the arterial-alveolar CO_2 difference.

Restrictive Lung Disease

Patients may develop reduced lung volumes (i.e., restrictive lung disease) as a result of diffuse interstitial pulmonary fibrosis, muscle weakness, or skeletal deformities. Patients with pulmonary fibrosis tend to exhibit an increased minute ventilation with small tidal volumes and an increased respiratory rate. This breathing pattern does not appear to be a result of hypercapnia or hypoxia and is unchanged by breathing 100% oxygen.[38] Although the mechanisms underlying this breathing pattern are unclear, they appear to be neural and related to mechanoreceptors in the chest wall. This is supported by observations in normals subjected to chest strapping.[39] The latter limitation of rib cage expansion appears to alter breathing in a fashion similar to interstitial lung disease. Both groups in fact showed higher levels of ventilation and occlusion pressure at elevated levels of CO_2, although the actual response slopes do not differ significantly from the normal state.[40] Thus, in contrast to the mechanical load imposed by airway resistance, the changes brought about by reduced chest wall and lung compliance do not produce a diminished ventilatory response to hypercapnia. Although there appear to be no data with respect to the hypoxic ventilatory response, the effects are likely to be similar.

In patients with restrictive disease associated with skeletal deformities, respiratory failure can develop as a result of their abnormal pulmonary function or diminished chemosensitivity or both. In scoliosis patients the reduction in the ventilatory responses to hypercapnia and hypoxia are totally related to the extent of pulmonary function abnormalities.[41, 42]

In the presence of neuromuscular disease the neural output of the respiratory center as reflected by occlusion pressure ($P_{0.1}$) tends to be unaffected, while the ventilatory response is decreased. This has been nicely characterized in normal volunteers during partial curarization.[43]

Obesity Hypoventilation Syndrome

Patients with obesity have a marked mechanical impediment in the form of an increased elastic load to breathing provided by the massive chest wall. Some obese patients also manifest hypoventilation, somnolence, erythrocytosis, and pulmonary hypertension as part of the obesity hypoventilation syndrome. These patients have blunted ventilatory responses to hypoxia and hypercapnia as a result of their intrinsic chemical sensitivity.[44] The extra mechanical load tends to facilitate hypoventilation in the face of the low respiratory responses. Treatment is therefore aimed at reducing the elastic load as well as administering respiratory stimulants. In obese patients with obstructive sleep apnea, therapy is also directed at relieving upper airway obstruction, since such patients do not compensate with increased neural drive in the face of upper airway obstruction.[45] Tracheostomy has been shown to restore CO_2 responsiveness to nearly normal in such patients.[46]

Metabolic and Endocrine Factors

Variations in metabolic rate have been shown to influence ventilatory responses. Increases in metabolic rate associated with hyperthermia or disease states such as hyperthyroidism augment ventilatory responses.[47] Similarly, in the disease states such as hypothyroidism the reduced metabolic rate is associated with depressed responses.[48] Starvation is also accompanied by a reduction in metabolic rate; indeed, semistarvation (i.e., caloric restriction to 500 to 600 calories daily) affected both hypoxic and hypercapneic responses.[49] It is interesting that such caloric intake would be that resulting from 3 liters of 5% dextrose in water.

In diabetes mellitus the autonomic neuropathy has been associated with defective cardiovascular and respiratory reflexes, including an increased incidence of sleep apnea.[50] Patients with diabetic neuropathy demonstrate disordered ventilatory control in the form of reduced response to hypercapnia and failure of hypoxia to augment the response to CO_2.[51] In diabetic patients without neuropathy, rate and ventilatory responses to hypoxia are blunted, but the response to hypercapnia appears to be preserved.[52]

In patients with cirrhosis of the liver hyperventilation and respiratory alkalosis are common and are often complicated by arterial hypoxemia. Although the response to CO_2 appears to be augmented at low levels of CO_2, at higher levels it is diminished.[53] The onset of liver failure appears to be associated with heightened sensitivity of peripheral chemoreceptors to hypoxia[54] but a diminution of the central response to CO_2.[55] The latter may be a function of the relative alkalosis in the cerebrospinal fluid. Chronic compensation tends to reduce pH back toward normal by decreasing bicarbonate. Thus the brain pH is less well defended against acute hypercapnia, and cerebral function may rapidly deteriorate.

REFERENCES

1. Peterson DD, Pack AI, Silage DA, Fishman AP. Effects of aging on ventilatory and occlusion pressure responses to hypoxia and hypercapnia. Am Rev Respir Dis 1981;124:287–391.

2. Kroneberg RS, Drage CW. Attenuation of the ventilatory and heart rate responses to hypoxia and hypercapnia with aging in normal men. J Clin Invest 1973;52:1812–1819.

3. Avery ME, Chernick V, Dutton RE, Permutt S. Ventilatory responses to inspired carbon dioxide in infants and adults. J Appl Physiol 1963;18:895–903.

4. Frantz ID, Adler SM, Thach BT, Taeusch HW. Maturational effects on respiratory response to carbon dioxide in premature infants. J Appl Physiol 1976;41:41–45.

5. Rigatto H, Torreverdusco R, Cates DB. Effects of O$_2$ on the ventilatory response to CO$_2$ in preterm infants. J Appl Physiol 1975;39:896–899.

6. Easton PA, Slykerman J, Anthonisen NR. Ventilatory response to sustained hypoxia in normal adults. J Appl Physiol 1986;61:906–911.

7. Schiffman PL, Westlake RE, Santiago TV, Edelman NH. Ventilatory control in parents of victims of sudden death syndrome. N Engl J Med 1980;320:486–491.

8. Mountain R, Zwillich C, Weil J. Hypoventilation in obstructive disease. The role of familial factors. N Engl J Med 1978;298:521–525.

9. Collins DD, Scoggin CH, Zwillich CW, Ewil JV. Hereditary aspects of decreased hypoxic drive in endurance athletes. J Appl Physiol 1978;44:464–468.

10. Lakshminaryan S, Pierson DJ. Recurrent high altitude pulmonary edema with blunted chemosensitivity. Am Rev Respir Dis 1975;11:869–872.

11. Schoene RB. Control of ventilation in climbers to extreme altitude. J Appl Physiol 1982;53:886–890.

12. Schoene RB, Lahiri S, Hackett PH, et al. The relationship of hypoxic ventilatory response to exercise performance on Mt. Everest. J Appl Physiol 1984;56:1478–1483.

13. Byrne-Quinn E, Sodal IE, Weil JV. Hypoxic and hypercapneic ventilatory drives in children native to high altitude. J Appl Physiol 1972;32:44–46.

14. Blesa MI, Lahiri S, Phil D, Rashkind W, Fishman AP. Normalization of the blunted ventilatory response to acute hypoxia in congenital cyanotic heart disease. N Engl J Med 1977;290:237–241.

15. Phillipson EA. Control of breathing during sleep. Am Rev Respir Dis 1978;118:909–939.

16. Douglas NJ, White DP, Weil JV, et al. Hypoxic ventilatory response decreases during sleep in normal men. Am Rev Respir Dis 1982;125:286–289.

17. Wasserman K, Whipp BJ, Koyal SN, Clearly MC. Effect of carotid body resection on ventilatory and acid-base control during exercise. J Appl Physiol 1975;39:354–358.

18. Martin BJ, Weil JV, Sparks KE, McCullough RE, Grover RF. Exercise ventilation correlates positively with ventilatory chemoresponsiveness. J Appl Physiol 1978;48:447–464.

19. Pernoll ML, Metcalfe J, Kovach PA, Wachtel R, Dunham MJ. Ventilation during rest and exercise in pregnancy and postpartum. Respir Physiol 1975;25:295–310.

20. England SJ, Fahri LE. Fluctuations in alveolar CO$_2$ and in base excess during the menstrual cycle. Respir Physiol 1976;26:157–161.

21. Schoene RB, Robertson T, Pierson DJ, Peterson AP. Respiratory drives and exercise in menstrual cycles of athletic and nonathletic women. J Appl Physiol 1981;50:1300–1305.

22. Vejby-Christiansen H, Petersen ES. Effect of body temperature and hypoxia on the ventilatory CO$_2$ response in man. Respir Physiol 1973;19:322–332.

23. Zwillich CW, Sahn SA, Weil JV. Effects of hypermetabolism on ventilation and chemosensitivity. J Clin Invest 1977;60:900–906.

24. Rodriguez JL, Askanazi J, Weissman C, Hensle TW, Rosenbaum SH, Kinney JM. Ventilatory and metabolic effects of glucose infusions. Chest 1985;88:512–518.

25. Brodsky JD, Macdonell JA, Cherniack RM. The respiratory response to carbon dioxide in health and emphysema. J Clin Invest 1960;39:724–729.

26. West JB. Causes of carbon dioxide retention in lung disease. N Engl J Med 1971;284:1232–1236.

27. Lourenco RV, Miranda JM. Drive and performance of the ventilatory apparatus in chronic obstructive lung disease. N Engl J Med 1968;279:53–59.

28. Gelb AF, Klein E, Schiffman P, Lugliani R, Aronstam P. Ventilatory response and drive in acute and chronic obstructive pulmonary disease. Am Rev Respir Dis 1977;116:9–16.

29. Fahey PJ, Hyde RW. "Won't breathe" vs "Can't breathe." Detection of depressed ventilatory drive in patients with obstructive pulmonary disease. Chest 1983;84:19–25.

30. Gelb AF, Klein E, Schiffman P, Lugliani R, Aronstam P. Ventilatory response and drive in acute and chronic obstructive pulmonary disease. Am Rev Respir Dis 1977;116:9–16.

31. Surli J, Grassino A, Lorange G, Milic-Emili J. Control of breathing in patients with chronic obstructive lung disease. Clin Sci Mol Med 1978;54:295–304.
32. Bradley CA, Fleetham JA, Anthonisen NR. Ventilatory control in patients with hypoxemia due to obstructive lung disease. Am Rev Respir Dis 1979;120:21–30.
33. Kepron W, Cherniack RM. The ventilatory response to hypercapnia and to hypoxemia in chronic obstructive lung disease. Am Rev Respir Dis 1973;108:843–850.
34. Bradley CA, Fleetham JA, Anthonisen NR. Ventilatory control in patients with hypoxemia due to obstructive lung disease. Am Rev Respir Dis 1979;120:21–30.
35. Aubier M, Murciano D, Fournier M, Milic-Emili J, Pariente R, Derenne J. Central respiratory drive in acute respiratory failure of patients with chronic obstructive lung disease. Am Rev Respir Dis 1980;122:191–199.
36. Aubier M, Murciano D, Milic-Emili J, et al. Effects of O_2 administration on ventilation and blood gases in acute respiratory failure of patients with chronic obstructive lung disease. Am Rev Respir Dis 1980;122:747–754.
37. Sassoon CSH, Hassell KT, Mahutte CK. Hyperoxic-induced hypercapnia in stable chronic obstructive pulmonary disease. Am Rev Respir Dis 1987;135:909–911.
38. Lourenco RV, Turino GM, Davidosn LAG, Fishman AP. The regulation of ventilation in diffuse pulmonary fibrosis. Am J Med 1965;38:199–216.
39. Dimarco AF, Kelsen SG, Cherniack NS, Hough WH, Bothe B. Effect on breathing of selective restriction of movement of the rib cage and abdomen. J Appl Physiol 1981;50:412–420.
40. Dimarco AJ, Kelsen SG, Cherniack NS, Bothe B. Occlusion pressure and breathing pattern in patients with interstitial lung disease. Am Rev Respir Dis 1983;127:425–430.
41. Kafer ER. Idiopathic scoliosis: mechanical properties of the respiratory system and the ventilatory response to carbon dioxide. J Clin Invest 1975;55:1151–1163.
42. Smyth RJ, Chapman KR, Wright TA, Crawford JS, Rebuch AS. Ventilatory patterns during hypoxia, hypercapnia, and exercise in adolescents with mild scoliosis. Pediatrics 1986;77:692–697.
43. Holle RHO, Schoene RB, Pavlin EJ. Effect of respiratory muscle weakness on $P_{0.1}$ induced by partial curarization. J Appl Physiol 1984;57:1150–1157.
44. Sharp J, Barrocas M, Chokroverty S. The cardiorespiratory effects of obesity. Clin Chest Med 1980;1:103–118.
45. Rajagopal KR, Abbrecht PH, Tellis CJ. Control of breathing in obstructive sleep apnea. Chest 1984;85:174–180.
46. Guilleminalt C, Cumminskey J. Progressive improvement of apnea index and ventilatory response to CO_2 after tracheostomy in obstructive sleep apnea syndrome. Am Rev Respir Dis 1982;126:14–20.
47. Engel LA, Ritchie B. Ventilatory response to inhaled carbon dioxide in hyperthyroidism. J Appl Physiol 1971;30:173–177.
48. Zwillich CW, Pierson DJ, Hofeldt FD, Lufkin EG, Weil JV. Ventilatory control in myxedema and hypothyroidism. N Engl J Med 1975;292:662–665.
49. Doekel RC, Willich CW, Scoggin CH, Kryger M, Weil JV. Clinical semistarvation. Depression of hypoxic ventilatory response. N Engl J Med 1976;295:358–361.
50. Rees PJ, Cochrane GM, Prior JG, Clark TJH. Sleep apnea in diabetic patients with autonomic neuropathy. J R Soc Med 1981;74:192–195.
51. Homma I, Kageyama S, Nagai T, Taniguchi I, Sakai T, Abe M. Chemosensitivity in patients with diabetic neuropathy. Clin Sci 1981;61:599–603.
52. Nishimura M, Miyamoto K, Suzuki A, Yamamoto H, Tsuji M, Kishi F. Ventilatory and heart rate responses to hypoxia and hypercapnia in patients with diabetes mellitus. Thorax 1989;44:251–257.
53. Karetzky MS, Mithoefer JC. The cause of hyperventilation and arterial hypoxia in patients with cirrhosis of the liver. Am J Med Sci 1967;254:797–804.
54. Stanley NN, Kelsen SG, Cherniack NS. Effect of liver failure on the ventilatory response to hypoxia in man and the goat. Clin Sci 1976;50:25–35.
55. Stanley NN, Salisbury BG, McHenry LC, Cherniac NS. Effect of liver failure on the response of ventilation and cerebral circulation to carbon dioxide in man and in the goat. Clin Sci 1975;49:157–169.

Chapter 6

Effects of Drugs on Respiratory Control

The vast majority of drugs used in the practice of anesthesiology such as analgesics, sedatives, hypnotics, and volatile anesthetic agents have as their principal side effect an alteration of respiratory control. This is manifested as a depressed desire to breathe. This chapter addresses the clinical relevance of these many drugs, whose effects may seriously impair ventilation in the perioperative period.

INHALATION ANESTHETICS

CO$_2$ Responses

Each of the halogenated inhalation agents currently in use (halothane, enflurane, and isoflurane) produces profound respiratory depression in a dose-related manner. This respiratory depression is far greater than that associated with older, outmoded agents (ether, cyclopropane, or fluroxene). At concentrations that produce loss of consciousness and surgical anesthesia, tidal volume is reduced. Although respiratory rate increases, minute ventilation decreases and an elevation of CO$_2$ occurs in proportion to the depth of anesthesia as a function of the minimum alveolar concentration (MAC). The extent of this hypoventilation and CO$_2$ retention varies with each agent. At 1.0 MAC halothane produces a modest increase in CO$_2$ to about 45 mm Hg. By comparison, the same level of isoflurane increases CO$_2$ to about 50 mm Hg, while enflurane produces even more marked hypercapnia to above 60 mm Hg.[1] While the effects of surgical stimulation tend to counteract this rise in CO$_2$, the hypercapnia tends to worsen in patients with chronic obstructive pulmonary disease (COPD) in proportion to their degree of airway obstruction.[2] In the face of the added mechanical load such patients are unable to achieve adequate gas exchange with the rapid, shallow breathing pattern associated with halothane.

94

The normal increase in ventilation with increasing CO_2 (i.e., the slope of the response) is blunted by the inhalation anesthetics in a dose-dependent manner. Whereas sedating halothane doses (0.1 MAC) produce little or no change in the slope of the response (Fig. 6.1), anesthetizing doses (1.0 MAC) produce significant decreases in slope. The observations of Tusiewicz et al.[3] indicate that much of this ventilatory depression is due to a reduction of rib cage recruitment that occurs at higher levels of ventilation in the awake state. The latter may also help to explain the effects of surgical stimulation, which produces a decrease in resting CO_2 but no change in the slope of the CO_2 response.[4]

Information about the role of mechanical factors in the reduced CO_2 response slope in humans is sketchy. Derenne et al.[5] studied a now obsolete agent, methoxyflurane, and noted that although the slope of the ventilatory response was decreased in the anesthetized state, the occlusion pressure response was minimally changed from the awake state. They suggested that much of the ventilatory depression was due to increased lung-thorax elastance and not reduced neural drive. With enflurane the role of mechanical factors appeared to be less dramatic. Wahba[6] concluded that both drive and timing appeared to be affected. Differences in respiratory timing also appear to account for some of the difference in respiratory depression between halothane and enflurane. The latter appears to be associated with a considerably slower breathing frequency.[7]

The absence of wakefulness with the inhalation anesthetics results in a complete dependence on the chemical regulation of ventilation. Thus, passive hyperventilation that removes the CO_2 stimulus results in apnea. Such apnea

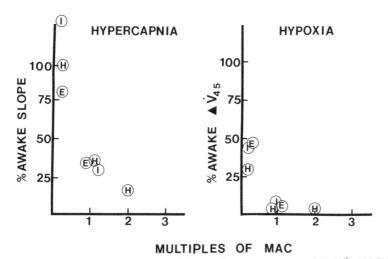

Figure 6.1. Relative changes in the slope of the ventilatory responses to CO_2 ($\Delta\dot{V}_E/\Delta CO_2$) and hypoxia ($\Delta\dot{V}_{45}$) resulting from sedating (0.1 MAC) and anesthetic concentrations of halothane (H), isoflurane (I), and enflurane (E). (Data are adapted from the work of Knill et al.[10–12])

is difficult if not impossible to elicit in conscious subjects but is easy to achieve during anesthesia. This CO_2 level, which is 5 to 9 mm Hg below the normal awake resting value, is referred to as the apneic threshold, a term coined by Fink and colleagues.[8] The apneic threshold can be estimated by linear extrapolation of the CO_2 response curve to zero ventilation (see *D* in Fig. 4.3).

Response to Hypoxia

Traditional views of the peripheral chemoreceptors considered them the body's last defense and resistant to drug depression. Present knowledge, however, recognizes that these structures are profoundly depressed in humans by even sedating levels of anesthesia (Fig. 6.1). The initial studies in dogs by Weiskopf and associates demonstrated blunting of the hypoxic response with 1.1% halothane.[9] Knill and Gelb[10] noted that depression of the response in humans was even more profound. Similar effects were seen with enflurane[11] and isoflurane.[12] Noteworthy is the relatively profound depression of the response in contrast to the hypercapneic response (Fig. 6.1). At levels that minimally affect the CO_2 response the hypoxic response is nearly abolished. This also appears to be true for nitrous oxide, which at concentrations of 30 to 50% has no effect on the CO_2 response but depresses the ventilatory response to hypoxia.[13] Furthermore, it has been shown in anesthetized humans[10] and dogs[9] that the normal synergistic interaction between hypoxia and hypercapnia is eliminated. Rather than acting to increase ventilation the two stimuli act to depress ventilation in anesthetized subjects.

Like the response to hypoxia the response to added $[H^+]$ to produce metabolic acidemia is mediated via peripheral chemoreceptors. Knill and associates[14] have shown that halothane sedation and anesthesia in humans markedly attenuates the response to acidemia and its attendant interaction with hypoxemia. Thus any patient compensation for these derangements must arise from measures instituted by the physician.

INTRAVENOUS ANESTHETICS

Barbiturates

Among the various CNS depressants used to achieve sedation, the barbiturates do not appear to have a significant effect on resting ventilation when used in doses that produce sedation or drowsiness. Intramuscular pentobarbital (2 mm/kg) reduced the ventilatory response to hypoxia in five of ten healthy volunteers for a period of about 90 minutes.[15] Sedative doses of thipental did not significantly affect resting ventilation or the response to isocapneic hypoxia and hyperoxic hypercapnia.[16] However, anesthetic levels of thiopental depressed both hypoxic and hypercapneic response to nearly the same extent (35 to 45% of control). In this respect the barbiturates differ from inhalation anesthetics, since the latter group depress hypoxic responses far in excess of their effects on hypercapneic responses.

Ketamine

The dissociative anesthetic ketamine appears to have minimal depressant actions on respiratory control. Early observations suggested that intravenous doses of 2.2 mg/kg did not affect resting ventilation or the response to CO_2 challenge.[17] In a study of dogs anesthetized with ketamine the hypercapneic response appeared to be increased,[18] and this led to speculation that ketamine may be a respiratory stimulant by virtue of the increased sympathetic nervous system activity. However, another more precisely controlled study in dogs demonstrated that ketamine produced slight but significant depression of both hypoxic and hypercapneic responses.[19] In healthy human volunteers 3 mg/kg ketamine administered intravenously appears to produce respiratory depression similar to that observed with premedicant doses of morphine (0.2 mg/kg).[20] In children an intravenous bolus dose of ketamine produced nearly a 40% decrease in the CO_2 response slope.[21] This transient response disappeared in 30 minutes while a continuous infusion was maintained. The respiratory depression in the latter "steady-state" infusion period was similar to that observed in adults,[20] namely a rightward shift of the CO_2 response curve but no change in the slope.

Lidocaine

The amide local anesthetic lidocaine has been widely used to control arrhythmias, to produce regional anesthesia, and as an adjunct in combination with other general anesthetics. Lidocaine administered as an intravenous bolus (1.5 mg/kg) caused a transient 50% decrease in the slope of the CO_2 ventilatory response.[22] In the same subjects lidocaine infusion increased the slope. Serum lidocaine concentrations during the infusion were about 3 μg/ml, a level similar to that seen after epidural block and similar to concentrations that produced up to a 28% reduction in anesthetic requirement.[23] These same steady-state lidocaine levels also produced depression of the hypoxic ventilatory response manifested by a 20% reduction in parameter A.[24]

SEDATIVES AND ATARACTICS

Benzodiazepines

The benzodiazepines have become increasingly popular as sedating agents and have virtually replaced barbiturates as preoperative medications, amnestic agents, and adjuvants to opioids. Intravenous doses of diazepam (0.1 to 0.4 mg/kg) have been shown to depress the slope of the CO_2 response.[25] This respiratory depression does not appear to be consistent in healthy subjects[26] or in patients with obstructive pulmonary disease.[27] Gross et al.[28] have clarified the transient nature of the response and have demonstrated that the depressant effect peaks in about 3 minutes and lasts for 30 minutes. More importantly, they showed that the ventilatory depression correlated with the subject's state of consciousness (Fig. 6.2). The effects of another benzodiazepine, midazolam, were qualitatively similar to those of diazepam with perhaps a slightly briefer duration of effect.[29]

The ventilatory response to hypoxia appears to be blunted by diazepam in a transient fashion and to a similar extent as the hypercapneic response. Lakshminarayan et al.[30] observed a decrease in parameter *A* to about one-half of control values in eight healthy volunteers. The effect was consistently demonstrated for 30 minutes after intravenous administration of 10 mg of diazepam.

Antagonism of the clinical effects of benzodiazepines (somnolence and respiratory depression) has not been totally reliable. Spaulding et al.[31] observed that physostigmine, a drug with central cholinergic activity, increased the level of consciousness but did not reverse the respiratory depression asso-

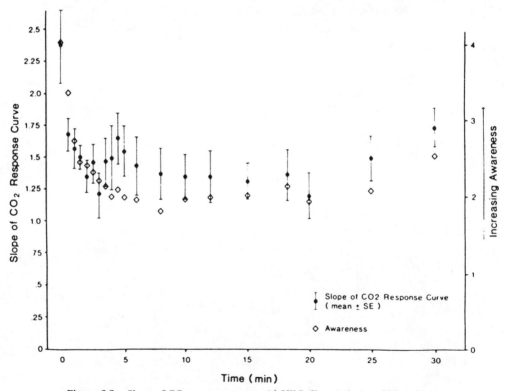

Figure 6.2. Slope of CO_2 response curves ($\pm$ SEM) (liters/min/mm Hg) and awareness scores during the 30 minutes following the intravenous injection of diazepam. (Reproduced with permission from Gross JB, Smith L, Smith TC. Time course of ventilatory response to carbon dioxide after intravenous diazepam. Anesthesiology 1982;57:18–21.)

ciated with diazepam. Recently, substances have been synthesized to produce direct antagonism of the effects of benzodiazepine. Of these, flumazenil (Ro 15-1788) has undergone clinical investigations. In healthy subjects intravenous administration promptly restored consciousness and orientation.[32] Despite this dramatic reversal of benzodiazepine-induced somnolence, there are no studies to date that clearly demonstrate reversal of respiratory depression.

Tranquilizers

Tranquilizer-type drugs such as phenothiazines, butyrophenones, and antihistamines have been used largely in hopes of potentiating the analgesia of narcotics. When used alone phenothiazines may cause slight but not significant depression of the CO_2 response and similar slight but inconsistent additive effects to narcotics.

Of particular interest to anesthesiologists is the butyrophenone droperidol, which was introduced as a compound to produce sedation and detachment from environmental stimuli and to act as an antiemetic in the presence of narcotics such as fentanyl. Droperidol does not appear to add to the depression of CO_2 responsiveness produced by fentanyl,[33, 34] nor does it consistently produce respiratory depression when used by itself in large doses (0.3 mg/kg I.V.).[35]

Recent interest has developed on the respiratory effects of droperidol and its relative haloperidol because of their effects on the hypoxic ventilatory response. Both compounds appear to be antagonists of dopamine. The latter appears to depress the hypoxic response in normal humans without affecting CO_2 response.[36] Complete block of this dopamine response is accomplished with haloperidol[37] and droperidol.[38] This antagonism of dopamine action at the peripheral chemoreceptor may explain why droperidol enhances the normal response to hypoxia[38] but does not affect the CO_2 response.[35]

OPIOIDS

The term "opiate" is usually reserved for compounds that are naturally derived from the opium poppy. These include morphine, codeine, and thebaine. The term "opioid" includes all drugs that are similar in structure or physiological effect to the most prominent naturally occurring compound, morphine. The extraction and purification of many natural compounds and the synthesis of many derivatives has resulted in a whole host of opioid compounds with pure agonist, pure antagonist, and mixed agonist-antagonist action.

Agonists

Morphine, the prototype of the pure opioid agonists, depresses ventilation in the usual analgesic doses (10 to 20 mg). This is manifested by a decrease in respiratory frequency, a small decrease in tidal volume, and a resultant increase in resting CO_2. The CO_2 response with such doses is altered primarily by a rightward displacement with little or no change in slope (Fig. 6.3). Larger doses of morphine (0.5 mg/kg) begin to depress the CO_2 response slope in a fashion that appears to be related to the depression in the state of consciousness. Indeed, sleep has been shown to enhance the ventilatory depression of morphine.[39] Other opioids consistently demonstrate the same pattern and degree of respiratory depression when given in equianalgesic doses. Much of the depression is mediated by depression of the contribution of the rib cage to ventilation.[40] This phenomenon is similar but less marked than that observed with halothane anesthesia.[3] However, the decrease in respiratory rate, in contrast to the tachypnea noted with halothane, results in a disproportionate decrease in minute ventilation.

The hypoxic response, much like with the inhalation anesthetics, was originally felt to be unaffected by opioids. However, depressed hypoxic responses have been demonstrated following administration of morphine (7.5 mg subcutaneously)[41] and meperidine (1.2 mg/kg orally).[42] Much like the benzodiazepines and barbiturates, but unlike the inhalation anesthetics, the magnitude of depression with opioids is approximately the same for both hypoxic and hypercapneic responses.

The safety of parenteral opioids is limited by the risk of severe ventilatory depression with increasing doses. Intrathecal and epidural administration of

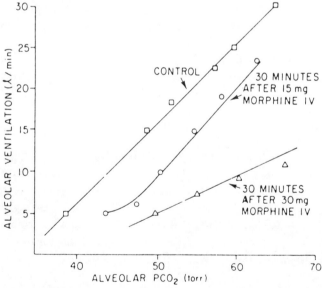

Figure 6.3.   Effects of morphine on the ventilatory response to CO_2. A typical premedicant dose (15 mg) is compared with a larger, more sedating dose (30 mg) likely to be associated with a greater decrease in the level of consciousness. (Reproduced with permission from Bailey PL, Stanley TH. Pharmacology of intravenous narcotic anesthetics. In: Miller RD, ed. Anesthesia. 3rd ed. New York: Churchill-Livingstone, 1990.)

opioids was initially felt to be free of such risk because relatively small doses are required to achieve high concentrations at the dorsal spinal roots, thereby obviating systemic toxicity. However, there is evidence that epidural administration of morphine produces respiratory depression of slightly greater magnitude than the same dose of drug administered parenterally.[43] The ventilatory depression is delayed and prolonged with the epidural administration and has been attributed to rostral spread of the drug along the neuraxis. With fentanyl the respiratory effects were also greater with epidural administration.[44] Since plasma fentanyl levels were lower in the epidural group, the authors also ascribed the effects to rostral spread despite the highly lipid-soluble character of fentanyl. In contrast, observations with another more lipid-soluble opioid, sufentanil, suggest that an important part of the analgesic and respiratory effects of that drug is also mediated centrally, but only after systemic absorption occurs.[45]

Antagonists

The opioid antagonists have been employed to reverse the ventilatory depression of the opioid agonists. The originally available compounds, nalorphine and levallorphan, possessed agonist as well as antagonist activity. Naloxone, the only pure antagonist available with no agonist activity, produces no effect in individuals who have not received an opioid. The drug must be given parenterally because of significant first-pass metabolism in the liver when given orally. Its major limitation is a short duration of action compared to most of the agonists it is used to reverse. A more potent, longer-acting derivative of naloxone, naltrexone, is available but only in oral form. Recently nalmefene, a naltrexone derivative with an even longer duration of action, has been developed. Pretreatment with intravenous nalmefene antagonized opioid challenge with fentanyl for more than 8 hours.[46] Furthermore, reversal of morphine-induced respiratory depression was sustained and not characterized by renarcotization as is the case with naloxone.[47]

Agonist-Antagonists

The drugs initially used to antagonize the effects of morphine possessed a mixed activity. When administered in the absence of a pure agonist they produced effects similar to the agonist drugs, namely analgesia, respiratory depression, and sedation. This agonist activity is rather weak and is characterized by a "ceiling effect"; i.e., a point at which increasing dose produces no increase in effect (Fig. 6.4). Approximate ceiling doses of agonist-antagonist compounds are listed in Table 6.1.

There has been a recent resurgence in the use of mixed agonist-antagonist opioids to reverse respiratory depression following high-dose opioid anesthesia and yet allow analgesia to persist. It is important to realize that the net effect of an agonist-antagonist opioid in a patient previously given a pure opioid ago-

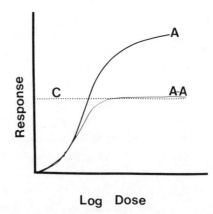

Figure 6.4. Diagrammatic dose-response relationships for a pure opioid agonist (*A*) and a typical agonist-antagonist (*A-A*) compound. Dotted line *C* indicates the "ceiling effect."

nist depends on how depressed the patient is to begin with. The interaction with a pure opioid agonist converges to a point that corresponds to the limited maximum effect or ceiling of the agonist-antagonist. If the existing effects of the agonist opioid at the time the agonist-antagonist opioid is given greatly exceed this ceiling effect, the agonist-antagonist will reverse the agonist by substituting its limited respiratory depression, analgesia, and sedation for the more marked effects of the agonist. If the agonist effect approximates the ceiling effect of the agonist-antagonist, little or no change will be noted after administration of the agonist-antagonist. Finally, if the agonist effect is less than the ceiling effect of the agonist-antagonist the analgesia and respiratory depression will actually increase.

The charcteristic respiratory depressant properties of the ceiling doses of mixed agonist-antagonists resemble those of premedicant doses (0.15 mg/kg) of morphine with respect to the ventilatory response to CO_2 (Fig. 6.3). Although there is scant information regarding the ventilatory sensitivity to hypoxia, the effects of the agonist-antagonists are likely to approximate those of morphine as well.[48]

Table 6.1.
Ceiling Doses of Opioid Agonist-Antagonists

Compound	Approximate Ceiling Doses[a]
	mg
Butorphanol	4
Dezocine	20
Nalbuphine	15
Nalorphine	50
Pentazocine	70

[a] Based on a 70-kg man.

ETHANOL

The central nervous system depression by alcohol resembles that produced by general anesthesia when an overdose occurs. At lower blood levels ethanol produces a dose-dependent rightward shift in the ventilatory response to CO_2.[49] A significant depression of the hypoxic ventilatory response also occurs[50] and raises the possibility that ethanol may play a role in the development of respiratory failure in patients with preexisting ventilatory impairment. The ethanol-induced depression of hypoxic drive is unaffected, but the depression of hypercapneic drive is reversed by naloxone.[51] The latter suggests an opiate-mediated mechanism for the respiratory depression.

NEUROMUSCULAR BLOCKING DRUGS

The ventilatory effect of muscle relaxants results primarily from their action at the neuromuscular junction since they have no effect on the chemosensitive areas of respiratory control. The diaphragm is the least affected, while expiratory muscles are extremely sensitive. However, the muscle groups most significantly compromised by relaxants are those of the upper airway.[52] The result is inability to swallow or clear secretions and a tendency for soft tissue collapse long before ventilatory volume is significantly affected.

With respiratory muscle weakness, ventilation at high levels of CO_2 is decreased such that the slope of the CO_2 response ($\Delta\dot{V}E/\Delta Pco_2$) tends to decrease. In spite of the weakness and decreased $\dot{V}E$, occlusion pressure ($P_{0.1}$) does not decrease at high levels of CO_2 and the slope of the occlusion pressure response ($\Delta P_{0.1}/\Delta Pco_2$) does not change.[53] This appears to indicate an intact central drive in one who simply cannot breathe because of the limitation imposed by muscle weakness.

REGIONAL ANESTHETIC TECHNIQUES

Regional anesthetics produce motor blockade but are also associated with systemic absorption of local anesthetic, which may affect the respiratory control mechanism. High thoracic epidural block (C_7–T_7) decreased the slope of the hypercapneic ventilatory response,[54] principally by eliminating the contribution of the inspiratory muscles of the rib cage. Lumbar epidural analgesia (T_7–T_{10}) appeared to have a stimulating effect on the ventilatory response to CO_2, which the authors attributed to the systemic effects of lidocaine.[55] A similar stimulating effect was observed following axillary block with bupivacaine.[56] On the other hand, intercostal nerve blockade (T_6–T_{12}), which produced similar motor block and lidocaine levels as with epidural lidocaine, produced no changes in CO_2 chemosensitivity.[57]

With spinal anesthesia the sensory and motor blockade is not complicated by systemic absorption of local anesthetics. Spinal anesthesia with 0.5% isobaric bupivacaine[58] and hyperbaric tetracaine[59] is associated with a decrease in resting CO_2 tension and an increase in the ventilatory response to CO_2. The latter is manifested by a leftward shift in the ventilatory and occlusion pressure response curves. The authors speculated that removal of chest wall afferent receptors by the spinal block produces an increased desire to breathe, which is sometimes accompanied by complaints of dyspnea.

RESPIRATORY STIMULANTS

Progesterone

Interest in progesterone as a respiratory stimulant arises out of the increase in ventilation observed during pregnancy and during the luteal phase of the menstrual cycle. Progesterone has been used for treatment of various disorders of hypoventilation. Studies in normal males indicate that the stimulation of ventilation occurs as a result of augmented responses to both hypoxia and hypercapnia.[60] Although the exact mechanism of stimulation is unknown, it does not appear to be related to increases in body temperature as a result of the metabolic effects of progesterone.[61]

Salicylates

The increased ventilation seen with salicylates appears to result from two separate mechanisms: first an increased metabolic rate and CO_2 production, and later a direct stimulation of the central nervous system.[62] Aspirin enhances the ventilatory response to CO_2, presumably by acting on the medullary chemoreceptors, since the effect is not altered by vagotomy or carotid body denervation in animals.[63] The ventilatory response to hypoxia is also increased by aspirin ingestion[62] and is most likely related to the increased metabolic rate, as in thyrotoxicosis and hyperthermia.

Methylxanthines

The action of methylxanthines (caffeine and aminophylline) as respiratory stimulants has long been recognized. Increases in minute ventilation and decreases in arterial CO_2 have been observed in normal humans after administration of caffeine or aminophylline.[64] Stroud et al.[65] reported that aminophylline (6 mg/kg) produced sufficient stimulation to counter the respiratory depression associated with 100 mg of meperidine, and by itself produced a leftward shift in the CO_2 ventilation curve. Other work in normals has failed to demonstrate an increase in the CO_2 response but demonstrated significant increases in hypoxic sensitivity (parameter A).[66] Although the actual mechanism is unclear, this augmented hypoxic response appears to be similar to that seen with increased metabolic activity such as seen with thyrotoxicosis, hyperthermia, or exercise. Aminophylline also offsets the decline in the increased ventilation associated with sustained hypoxia.[67] This action has been attributed to its role as an adenosine blocker, since the neurotransmitter adenosine has a depressant effect on neural activity in many areas of the central nervous system.

Doxapram

Doxapram is a ventilatory stimulant that has been used in respiratory failure and has been suggested as a reversal for ventilatory depression from a wide variety of drugs. Although it possesses the nonspecific effect of increasing wakefulness, the major site of ventilatory stimulation appears to be at the peripheral chemoreceptors.[68] However, studies in normal subjects[69, 70] have demonstrated an increase in the ventilatory response to isocapneic hypoxia and to hyperoxic hypercapnia. The increased CO_2 responsiveness implies that doxapram has some central action.

The clinical effects of I.V. doxapram are rather evanescent (<10 minutes) and necessitate continuous infusion of drug. Nevertheless, the drug has often been touted as useful postoperatively to increase ventilation and speed elimination of inhalation anesthetics. However, the residual levels of the anesthetics profoundly depress the response to hypoxia and attenuate the increase in ventilation produced by doxapram,[10] presumably by their profound effects on the peripheral chemoreceptors.

Almitrine

Unlike doxapram, almitrine bismesylate, a triazine derivative, appears to be a specific stimulant to the peripheral chemoreceptors. Thus the drug increases the ventilatory response to hypoxia in humans but has little effect on the CO_2 response.[71] In patients with chronic airway obstruction almitrine increases Pao_2 and decreases $Paco_2$ as a result of the enhanced hypoxic ventilatory response and improved matching of ventilation and perfusion. The latter appears to be the result of enhanced hypoxic pulmonary vasoconstriction (HPV).[72] This same effect on HPV has also been demonstrated in normals.[73]

Inhalation anesthetics such as halothane profoundly depress the ventilatory response to hypoxia. Infusion of almitrine (0.5 mg/kg) appears to restore the hypoxic ventilatory drive and the peripheral chemosensitivity in halothane-anesthetized subjects.[74] Whether or not such therapy with almitrine in the postanesthetic recovery room is feasible remains to be seen.

REFERENCES

1. Hickey RF, Severinghaus JW. Regulation of breathing: drug effects in lung biology in health and disease. In: Hornbein TF, ed. Regulation of breathing. New York: Marcel Dekker, 1978;125:1312.
2. Pietak S, Weening CS, Hickey RF, Fairley HB. Anesthetic effects on ventilation in patients with chronic obstructive pulmonary disease. Anesthesiology 1975;42:160–166.

3. Tusiewicz KA, Bryan AC, Froese AB. Contributions of changing rib cage diaphragm interactions to the ventilatory depression of halothane anesthesia. Anesthesiology 1977;47:327–337.

4. Lam AM, Clement JL, Knill RL. Surgical stimulation does not enhance ventilatory chemoreflexes during enflurane anesthesia in man. Can Anaesth Soc J 1980;27:22–28.

5. Derenne JP, Couture J, Iscoe S, Whitelaw WA. Occlusion pressures in men rebreathing CO_2 under methoxyflurane anesthesia. J Appl Physiol 1976;40:805–814.

6. Wahba WM. Analysis of ventilatory depression by enflurane during clinical anesthesia. Anesth Analg 1980;59:103–109.

7. Byrick RJ, Janssen EG. Respiratory waveform and rebreathing in T-piece circuits: a comparison of enflurane and halothane waveforms. Anesthesiology 1980;53:371–378.

8. Hanks EC, Ngai SH, Fink BR. The respiratory threshold during halothane anesthesia. Anesthesiology 1961;22:393–397.

9. Weiskopf RB, Raymond LW, Severinghaus JW. Effects of halothane on canine respiratory response to hypoxia with and without hypercarbia. Anesthesiology 1974;41:350–360.

10. Knill RC, Gelb AW. Ventilatory responses to hypoxia and hypercapnia during halothane sedation and anesthesia in man. Anesthesiology 1978;49:244–251.

11. Knill RL, Manninen PH, Clement JL. Ventilation and chemoreflexes during enflurane sedation and anesthesia in man. Can Anaesth Soc J 1979;26:353–360.

12. Knill RL, Kieraszewicz HT, Dodgson BG. Chemical regulation of ventilation during isoflurane sedation and anaesthesia in humans. Can Anaesth Soc J 1983;30:607–614.

13. Yacoub O, Doell D, Dryger MH, Anthonisen NR. Depression of hypoxic ventilatory response by nitrous oxide. Anesthesiology 1976;45:385–389.

14. Knill RL, Clement JL. Ventilatory responses to acute metabolic acidemia in humans awake, sedated, and anesthetized with halothane. Anesthesiology 1985;62:745–753.

15. Hirshman CA, McCullough RE, Cohen PJ, Weil J. Effect of pentabarbitone on hypoxic ventilatory drive in man. Br J Anaesth 1975;47:963–968.

16. Knill RL, Bright S, Manninen P. Hypoxic ventilatory responses during thiopentone sedation and anesthesia in man. Can Anaesth Soc J 1978;25:366–372.

17. Virtue RW, Alanis JM, Mori M, LaFargue RT, Vogel JHK, Metcalf DR. An anesthetic agent: 2-orthochlorophenyl-2 methylamino cyclohexanone. MCI (CI-581). Anesthesiology 1967;28:823–833.

18. Soliman MG, Brindle GF, Kuster G. Response to hypercapnia under ketamine anesthesia. Can Anaesth Soc J 1975;22:486–494.

19. Hirshman CA, McCullough RE, Cohen PJ, Weil J. Hypoxic ventilatory drive in dogs during thiopental, ketamine, or pentobarbital anesthesia. Anesthesiology 1975;43:628–634.

20. Bourke DL, Malit LA, Smith TC. Respiratory interactions of ketamine and morphine. Anesthesiology 1987;66:153–157.

21. Hamza J, Ecoffey C, Gross JB. Ventilatory response to CO_2 following intravenous ketamine in children. Anesthesiology 1989;70:422–425.

22. Gross JB, Caldwell CB, Shaw LM, Laucks SO. The effect of lidocaine on the ventilatory response to carbon dioxide. Anesthesiology 1983;59:521–529.

23. Himes RS, DiFazio CA, Burney RG. Effects of lidocaine on the anesthetic requirements for nitrous oxide and halothane. Anesthesiology 1977;47:437–440.

24. Gross JB, Caldwell CB, Shaw LM, Apfelbaum JL. The effect of lidocaine infusion on the ventilatory response to hypoxia. Anesthesiology 1984;61:662–665.

25. Forster A, Gardaz JP, Suter PM, Gemperle M. Respiratory depression by midazolam and diazepam. Anesthesiology 1980;53:494–497.

26. Catchglove RF, Kafer EB. The effects of diazepam on ventilatory response to carbon dioxide and steady state gas exchange. Anesthesiology 1971;34:91–93.

27. Catchglove RF, Kafer EF. The effects of diazepam on respiration in patients with obstructive pulmonary disease. Anesthesiology 1971;34:14–18.

28. Gross JB, Smith L, Smith TC. Time course of ventilatory response to carbon dioxide after intravenous diazepam. Anesthesiology 1982;57:18–21.

29. Forster A, Gardaz JP, Suter PM, Gemperle M. Respiratory depression by midazolam and diazepam. Anesthesiology 1980;53:494–497.

30. Lakshminarayan S, Sahn S, Hudson LD, Weil JV. Effect of diazepam on ventilatory responses. Clin Pharmacol Ther 1976;20:178–183.

31. Spaulding BC, Choi SD, Gross JB, Apfelbaum JL, Broderson H. The effect of physotigmine on diazepam-induced ventilatory depression: a double-blind study. Anesthesiology 1984;61:551–554.

32. Lauven PM, Schwilden H, Stoeckel H, Greenblatt DJ. The effects of benzodiazepine antagonist Ro 15-1788 in the presence of stable concentration of midazolam. Anesthesiology 1985;63:61–64.

33. Kallos T, Smith TC. The respiratory effects of innovar given for premedication. Br J Anaesth 1969;41:303–306.

34. Harper MH, Hickey RF, Cromwell TH, Linwood S. The magnitude and duration of respiratory depression produced by fentanyl and fentanyl plus droperidol in man. J Pharmacol Exp Ther 1976;199:464–468.

35. Prokocimer P, Delavault E, Rey F, Lefevre P, Mazze RI, Desmonts JM. Effects of droperidol on respiratory drive in humans. Anesthesiology 1983;59:113–116.

36. Welsh MJ, Heistad DD, Abboud FM. Depression of ventilation by dopamine in man. J Clin Invest 1978;61:708–713.

37. Bainbridge CW, Heistad DD. Effect of haloperidol on ventilatory responses to dopamine in man. J Pharmacol Exp Ther 1980;213:13–17.

38. Ward DS. Stimulation of hypoxic ventilatory drive by droperidol. Anesth Analg 1984;63:106–110.

39. Forrest WH Jr, Belleville JW. The effect of sleep plus morphine on the respiratory response to carbon dioxide. Anesthesiology 1964;25:137–141.

40. Rigg JRA, Rondi P. Change in rib cage and diaphragm contribution to ventilation after morphine. Anesthesiology 1981;55:507–514.

41. Weil JV, McCullough RE, Kline JS, Sodal IE. Diminished ventilatory response to hypoxia and hypercapnia after morphine in normal man. N Engl J Med 1975;292:1103–1106.

42. Kryger MH, Yacoub O, Dosman J, Macklein PT, Anthonisen NR. Effect of meperidine on occlusion pressure responses to hypercapnia and hypoxia with and without external resistance. Am Rev Respir Dis 1976;114:333–340.

43. Knill RL, Clement JL, Thompson WR. Epidural morphine causes delayed and prolonged ventilatory depression. Can Anaesth Soc J 1981;28:537–543.

44. Negre I, Gueneron JP, Ecoffey C, Penon C, Gross JB, Levron JC, Samili K. Ventilatory response to carbon dioxide after intramuscular and epidural fentanyl. 1987;66:707–710.

45. Koren G, Sandler AN, Klein J, Whiting WC, Lau LC, Slavchenko P, Daley D. Relationship between the pharmacokinetics and the analgesic and respiratory pharmacodynamics of epidural sufentanil. Clin Pharmacol Ther 1989;46:455–462.

46. Gal TJ, DiFazio CA. Prolonged antagonism of opioid action with intravenous nalmefene in man. Anesthesiology 1986;64:175–180.

47. Konieczko KM, Jones JG, Arrowcliffe MP, Jordan C, Altman DG. Antagonism of morphine-induced respiratory depression with nalmefene. 1988;61:318–323.

48. Camporesi EM, Glass P, Moon RE, Steinhause E, Wagoner R. Ventilatory sensitivity to hypoxia after administration of an agonist-antagonist. Anesthesiology 1987;67:A541.

49. Johnstone RE, Rier CE. Acute respiratory effects of ethanol in man. Clin Pharmacol Ther 1973;14:501–508.

50. Sahn SA, Lakshminarayan S, Pierson DJ, Lieil JV. Effect of ethanol on the ventilatory response to oxygen and carbon dioxide in man. Clin Sci Mol Med 1974;49:33–38.

51. Michiels TM, Light RW, Mahutte K. Naloxone reverses ethanol-induced depression of hypercapneic drive. Am Rev Respir Dis 1983;128:823–826.

52. Dodgson BG, Knill RL, Clement JL. Curare increases upper airway resistance while reducing ventilatory muscle strength. Can Anaesth Soc J 1981;28:505–506.

53. Holle RHO, Schoene RB, Pavlin EJ. Effect of respiratory muscle weakness on $P_{0.1}$ induced by partial curarization. J Appl Physiol 1984;57:1150–1157.

54. Koch T, Sako S, Nishino T, Mizuguchi T. Effect of high thoracic extradural anesthesia on the ventilatory response to hypercapnia in normal volunteers. Br J Anaesth 1989;62:362–367.

55. Labaille T, Clergue F, Samii K, Ecoffey C, Berdeaux A. Ventilatory response to CO_2 following intravenous and epidural lidocaine. Anesthesiology 1985;63:179–183.

56. Negre I, Labaille T, Samii K, Noviant Y. Ventilatory response to CO_2 following axillary blockade with bupivacaine. Anesthesiology 1985;63:401–403.

57. Hecker BR, Bjurstrom R, Schoene RB. Effect of intercostal nerve blockade on respiratory mechanics and CO_2 chemosensitivity at rest and exercise. Anesthesiology 1989;70:131–138.
58. Steinbrook RA, Concepcion M, Topulos GP. Ventilatory responses to hypercapnia during bupivacaine spinal anesthesia. Anesth Analg 1988;67:247–252.
59. Steinbrook RA, Concepcion M. Ventilatory responses to hypercapnia during tetracaine spinal anesthesia. J Clin Anesth 1988;1:75–80.
60. Schoene RB, Pierson DJ, Lakshminarayan, Shrader DL, Butler J. Effect of medroxy progesterone acetate on respiratory drives and occlusion pressure. Clin Respir Physiol 1980;16:645–653.
61. Skatrud J, Dempsey JA, Daiser DJ. Ventilatory response to medroxy progesterone acetate in normal subjects: time course and mechanism. J Appl Physiol 1978;44:939–944.
62. Riley DJ, Legawiec BA, Santiago TV, Edelman NH. Ventilatory responses to hypercapnia and hypoxia during continuous aspirin ingestion. J Appl Physiol 1977;43:971–976.
63. Tenney SM, Miller RM. The respiratory and circulatory action of salicylate. Am J Med 1955;19:498–508.
64. Richmond CH. Action of caffeine and aminophylline as respiratory stimulants in man. J Appl Physiol 1949;2:16–20.
65. Stroud MW, Lambertsen CJ, Ewing R, Lough RH, Gould RA, Schmidt CG. Effects of aminophylline and mederidine alone and in combination on the respiratory response to carbon dioxide. J Pharmacol Exp Ther 1955;114:461–469.
66. Lakshminarayan S, Sahn SA, Weil JV. Effect of aminophylline on ventilatory responses in normal man. Am Rev Respir Dis 1978;117:33–38.
67. Easton PA, Anthonisen NR. Ventilatory response to sustained hypoxia after pretreatment with aminophylline. J Appl Physiol 1988;64:1455–1450.
68. Mitchell RA, Herbert DA. Potencies of doxapram and hypoxia in stimulating carotid-body chemoreceptors and ventilation in anesthetized cats. Anesthesiology 1975;42:559–566.
69. Calverley PMA, Robson RH, Wraith PK, Prescott LF, Flenley DC. The ventilatory effects of doxapram in normal man. Clin Sci 1983;650:65–69.
70. Burki NK. Ventilatory effects of doxapram in conscious human subjects. Chest 1984;85:600–604.
71. Stradling JR, Barnes P, Pride NB. The effects of almitrine on the ventilatory response to hypoxia and hypercapnia in normal subjects. Clin Sci 1982;63:401–404.
72. Connaughton JJ, Douglas NJ, Morgan AD, et al. Almitrine improves oxygenation when both awake and asleep in patients with hypoxia and carbon dioxide retention caused by chronic bronchitis and emphysema. Am Rev Respir Dis 1985;132:206–210.
73. Melot C, Dechamps P, Hallemans R, Decroly P, Mols P. Enhancement of hypoxic pulmonary vasoconstriction by low dose-almitrine bismesylate in normal humans. Am Rev Respir Dis 1989;139:111–119.
74. Clergue F, Ecoffey C, Derenne JP, Viars P. Oxygen drive to breathing halothane anesthesia: effects of almitrine bismesylate. Anesthesiology 1984;60:125–131.

SECTION III

Blood Flow and Gas Exchange

Chapter 7

Pulmonary Circulation

The primary function of the pulmonary circulation is respiratory, i.e., the transport of mixed venous blood through the alveolar capillaries so that gas exchange can be accomplished. This chapter deals primarily with the gas exchange function and considers the mechanisms that regulate the volume and distribution of blood flow. Initially, however, some of the non–gas exchange functions of the pulmonary circulation are briefly discussed.

NONRESPIRATORY FUNCTIONS

The lung is exposed to virtually the entire blood volume during a single circulation. The pulmonary circulation therefore can provide a protective function by acting as a filter to trap platelet aggregates, thrombi, and other debris. This can occur in some vessels while the remaining areas continue to perform gas exchange functions.

The pulmonary vessels are highly distensible and ordinarily contain about 10% of the total circulating blood volume. As such they also serve as a reservoir of blood for the left ventricle and allow left ventricular stroke volume to be maintained for several beats should pulmonary artery outflow be occluded.

In addition to transporting substances such as surfactant, for the lung's own use, the pulmonary circulation also carries chemicals activated or released in the lungs on to the blood stream to exert their effects in distant organs (Table 7.1). The pulmonary vessels also partake in the lung's complex system for clearing and modifying a variety of familiar compounds (Table 7.2), most of which are basic amines (pK > 8) of high lipid solubility.

PRESSURE-FLOW RELATIONSHIPS IN THE PULMONARY CIRCULATION

The pulmonary circulation resembles its systemic counterpart in that it has a pump, the right ventricle. It also has an exchange system (capillaries) inter-

Table 7.1.
Substances Released by the Lung

Angiotensin
Adenosine
Heparin
Histamine
Leukotrienes
Plasminogen activator
Prostacyclin
Serotonin

posed between the distributing system (pulmonary arteries and arterioles) and the collecting system (pulmonary veins). The pulmonary circulation differs from the systemic circuit because of the relatively low pressure within its vessels (Table 7.3), despite the fact that the lung receives a higher blood flow than any other organ since it must accept the entire cardiac output. Thus, in contrast to the systemic circuit with its high pressure and high resistance, the pulmonary circulation may be characterized as a high-flow, low-pressure, low-resistance system. This high-flow, low-pressure relationship exists not only at rest but even with exercise. The pulmonary circuit can accommodate a threefold to fourfold increase in cardiac output with only minimal increases in pulmonary artery pressure, largely because the thinner pulmonary vessels contain less smooth muscle and are more distensible than their systemic counterparts. The systemic vessels regulate blood flow to various organs, some of which lie above heart level. The pulmonary vessels, on the other hand, must always accept the entire cardiac output.

Distribution of Pulmonary Blood Flow

Relationships to Extravascular Pressure. The pulmonary arteries and veins within the lung parenchyma are surrounded by sheaths of connective tissue that serve as attachments for the alveolar walls. Thus when the subatmo-

Table 7.2.
Exogenous Substances Modified in the Lung

Amphetamine
Bupivacaine
Chlorpromazine
Diphenhydramine
Fentanyl
Imipramine
Lidocaine
Meperidine
Methadone
Procainamide
Propranolol

Table 7.3.
Hemodynamic Comparisons of Pulmonary and Systemic Circulation

	Pulmonary	Systemic
Arterial pressure, mm Hg		
systolic/diastolic	25/8	125/80
mean	12	95
Mean atrial pressure, mm Hg	5 (left)	2 (right)
Mean capillary pressure, mm Hg	6–10	18–25
Blood flow, liters/min	5	5
Blood volume, ml	400–500	5000–6000
Vascular resistance, mm Hg/	1.4[a]	18.6[a]
liter/min		

[a]To convert to CGS units (dyne · sec · cm^{-5}), multiply by 80.

spheric pleural pressure acts on the outer surface of the lung to produce lung expansion, an outward radial traction is exerted on the vessel sheaths and serves to increase vessel diameter (Fig. 7.1). These vessels are termed extraalveolar and include most arteries and veins larger than 30 μm in diameter. Other smaller vessels lie in and around the alveolar septae and are thus referred to as alveolar vessels. These vessels are exposed to alveolar pressure, and their caliber is determined by the relationships between the pressure within them and the surrounding alveolar pressure. Thus they are compressed in the presence of high alveolar pressures such as those associated with lung volume expansion (Fig. 7.1). While the resistance of the extraalveolar vessels decreases with lung expansion, the alveolar vessels undergo compression and

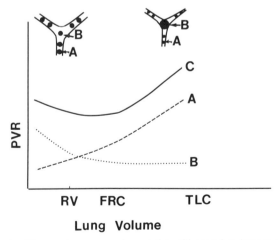

Figure 7.1. Effects of lung volume expansion on the caliber and resistance of the alveolar (*A*) and extraalveolar (*B*) pulmonary vessels. Note that the net effect on total resistance (*C*) results in the lowest value at functional residual capacity (FRC). Values for *C* increase toward residual volume (RV) and total lung capacity (TLC).

reduction in caliber, which increases their resistance. The net effect on both types of vessels results in a total pulmonary vascular resistance that is lowest at functional residual capacity (Fig. 7.1) and increases toward both extremes of lung volume.

Stratification of Blood Flow–Hemodynamic Zones.   Within the lung considerable inequality of blood flow exists. The use of radioactive xenon has demonstrated the topographic distribution of pulmonary blood flow. In the upright position blood flow decreases linearly from the bottom to the top of the lung such that flow at the apex is minimal. This uneven distribution has been attributed to hydrostatic pressure differences within the blood vessels arising from the effects of gravity. Thus the low-pressure pulmonary circuit appears barely able to raise a column of blood to the lung apex. This somewhat simplistic gravity-oriented explanation has been challenged by Badeer,[1] who attributes the decreased apical blood flow to increased vascular resistance. The gravitational pressure at the apex significantly lowers the intravascular and hence the transmural pressure of the highly compliant pulmonary vessels. As a result, they collapse and increase their resistance to flow. The distribution of pulmonary blood flow is governed chiefly by the distensibility of vessels and their transmural distending pressure. Because of the vertical gradient of pressure in this low-pressure system, several zones have been described in an effort to characterize the hemodynamic conditions that govern flow. West and his colleagues[2] have described these zones on the basis of the relationships between pressures in the pulmonary artery (Ppa), alveolus (Palv), and pulmonary vein (Pv). These relationships are summarized in Table 7.4.

In zone 1, which corresponds to the lung apices in the upright posture, alveolar pressure (Palv) is greater than pulmonary artery (Ppa) and pulmonary venous (Pv) pressures. This results in a decreased transmural pressure and virtual collapse of these vessels, which receive very little or no blood flow. Farther down the lung in zone 2 the Ppa increases and exceeds Palv, but Palv still exceeds Pv. Resistance to blood flow in this zone is therefore governed by the difference between Ppa and Palv and has been variously described as a vascular waterfall or a Starling resistor.

In zone 3 both Ppa and Pv exceed Palv, and blood flow is determined by the more conventional arterial to venous pressure gradient. This gradient is

Table 7.4.
Hemodynamic Zones of the Lung as Described by West et al.[2]

Zone	Pressure Relationships	Vessel Behavior	Determinant of Flow
1	Palv > Ppa > Pv	Collapsed	Little or no flow
2	Ppa > Palv > Pv	Starling resistor ("waterfall")	Ppa − Palv
3	Ppa > Pv > Palv	Distended	Ppa − Pv

constant throughout zone 3 and suggests that blood flow is constant throughout this zone, rather than continuing to increase toward more dependent lung zones. In reality, however, blood flow does increase toward the bottom of zone 3 because the transmural or distending pressure across vessel walls increases due to increases in Ppa and Pv, while Palv does not change. This progressive distending force serves to lower resistance to blood flow through the vessels of zone 3. If other extrinsic factors are present to cause narrowing of these vessels, resistance to blood flow in these dependent regions may increase and an additional area (zone 4) may exist in which the Ppa, Pv, and Palv relationships are the same as in zone 3 but blood flow is decreased.

The zonal distribution of blood flow based on the relationships of Ppa, Pv, and Palv provides a conceptual framework for understanding the nature of pulmonary blood flow distribution. However, these relationships do not account for all of the changes in blood flow distribution such as those associated with differing degrees of lung inflation. The vertical gradient of blood flow described in the zonal model is most pronounced at total lung capacity, i.e., after a maximal inspiration. The gradient is actually reversed after maximal expiration to residual volume. Since relationships between Ppa, Pv, and Palv remain relatively unchanged, other mechanical factors that affect vascular caliber must be invoked. These most likely represent changes in perivascular pressure and the influence of lung expansion on extraalveolar vessels.[3]

Pulmonary Vascular Resistance

The resistance to blood flow through the pulmonary circuit, pulmonary vascular resistance (PVR), is determined by the difference between the inflow pressure in the pulmonary artery (Ppa) and the outflow pressure or left atrial pressure (Pla). The ratio of this pressure drop across the pulmonary circuit to the total pulmonary blood flow ($\dot{Q}$), or cardiac output, is defined as PVR. The calculation of PVR provides information about the state of the pulmonary vasculature. When PVR is increased it is generally assumed, as in other vascular beds, that the pulmonary vessels are constricted. However, in the lung the situation is more complex because of such factors as lung inflation, the collapsibility of vessels, and hydrostatic forces that alter the interpretations of PVR.

Partitioning of Pulmonary Vascular Resistance.   A variety of techniques have been used to assess the distribution of pulmonary vascular resistance. However, there is still much uncertainty about the relative partition of resistance among the vessels that make up the pulmonary circuit. Clinically, the measurement of pulmonary artery occlusion pressure (PAOP) has been used to estimate left atrial pressure and also pulmonary capillary pressure (Pc). These latter two pressures are only the same if postcapillary or venous resistance is negligible. Nevertheless, under most normal conditions this venous resistance may contribute about 40% of total PVR.[4]

Total PVR can be calculated as

$$PVR = \frac{Ppa - PAOP}{CO}$$

Where PAOP is an estimate of left atrial pressure; CO is cardiac output; and Ppa is mean pulmonary artery pressure.

This total PVR can in turn be divided into two components: a precapillary or pulmonary arterial resistance (Ra) and a postcapillary or venous resistance (Rv).

$$Ra = \frac{Ppa - Pc}{CO}$$

$$Rv = \frac{Pc - PAOP}{CO}$$

Although it is not possible to measure pulmonary capillary pressure (Pc) in intact animals or patients, Holloway et al.[5] have developed a technique that uses pulmonary artery occlusion curves to derive Pc and thus estimate the components of PVR. The declining Ppa profile after balloon occlusion of a large pulmonary artery changes to a slower rate as blood spreads throughout the larger cross-sectional area of capillaries, veins, and left atrium. The inflection point from fast to slow (Fig. 7.2) is thought to represent Pc, and the difference between Pc and PAOP reflects the postcapillary or venous resistance (Rv). Although PAOP is often used clinically to estimate what is termed "pulmonary

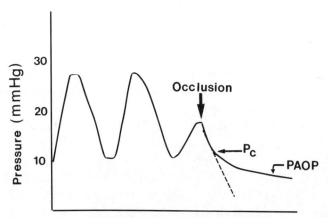

Figure 7.2.   Diagrammatic representation of the pulmonary artery pressure (Ppa) trace during balloon occlusion *(arrow)* to estimate pulmonary capillary pressure (Pc). PAOP, pulmonary artery occlusion pressure. The point at which the pressure trace deviates from the straight dashed line corresponds to Pc.

Table 7.5.
Factors That Actively Alter Pulmonary Vascular Resistance

Constrictors	Dilators
Sympathetic stimulation	Isoproterenol
Hypoxia	Acetylcholine
Hypercapnia	Bradykinin
Acidemia	Prostaglandins (E_1, I_2)
Catecholamines	Theophylline
Histamine (H_1)	
Serotonin	
Angiotensin II	
Prostaglandins (D_2, E_2, F_2, H_2)	
Substance P	

capillary wedge pressure," PAOP is not a capillary pressure and thus tends to underestimate Pc whenever PVR is increased as a result of changes in Rv.

Factors That Alter Pulmonary Vascular Resistance.   Changes in PVR may be classified as active or passive. Active changes imply pulmonary vasoconstriction and presuppose that no passive changes have occurred. Table 7.5 lists some neurogenic chemical and humoral factors that actively alter pulmonary vascular resistance. For the most part these vasoactive agents have similar effects on systemic as well as pulmonary vessels. One of the most obvious exceptions, however, is histamine. This is a vasodilator in the systemic circuit, whereas in the pulmonary circulation it produces vasoconstriction.

Passive changes in PVR imply that vessel caliber changes in response to factors such as lung mechanics or hemodynamics. Several such factors are listed in Table 7.6. It is difficult to identify the precise contribution of each of the factors, since many are interrelated so that a change in one effects a change in another, e.g., Pla and Ppa.

One remarkable characteristic of the low-pressure pulmonary circuit is its capacity to decrease PVR as pressure within the system, either venous or arterial, rises. Two mechanisms have been described to explain this: recruitment and distention. Recruitment reflects a reserve capacity of the capillary bed, which under normal conditions has some vessels essentially closed. As pressure

Table 7.6.
Factors That Passively Alter Pulmonary Vascular Resistance

Increased PVR	Decreased PVR
Lung inflation or deflation from FRC	Increased cardiac output
Increased perivascular pressure	Increased Ppa
	Increased Pla
Increased blood viscosity	Increased pulmonary blood volume

increases, these vessels open and blood flow is conducted through a vascular bed of greater cross-sectional area, thus lowering PVR. Most data indicate recruitment to be the primary mechanism for the decrease in PVR as pulmonary artery pressure increases above its normally low values. Further pressure increases result in distention of vessels that are open in response to the increase in perfusion. Thus distention appears to contribute to the decrease in PVR associated with higher intravascular pressures.

Another unique feature of the pulmonary circulation is that vessels are exposed to different distending forces as lung volume expands and contracts above and below functional residual capacity (Fig. 7.1). As a result, the caliber and length of the vessels (and hence their resistance) is passively governed by changes in lung volume. At low lung volumes (below FRC) the extraalveolar vessels are compressed and offer increased resistance to flow, which diminishes as lung volume is increased. Although the extraalveolar vessels are maximally expanded at high lung volumes and offer low resistance to flow, alveolar vessels offer increased resistance, since they become stretched and compressed.

HYPOXIC PULMONARY VASOCONSTRICTION

In the systemic vascular beds hypoxia produces vasodilation to aid oxygen delivery and carbon dioxide removal. The pulmonary vessels, on the other hand, respond to acute hypoxia by constricting. This unique behavior in response to hypoxia is called hypoxic pulmonary vasoconstriction (HPV). This HPV response is an important compensatory mechanism that serves to divert flow away from hypoxic alveoli. Blood flow thus shifts from poorly ventilated alveoli to better ventilated ones to match ventilation and perfusion and minimize arterial hypoxemia.

This physiological manifestation of HPV depends heavily on the size of the lung area that is hypoxic. If the segment of hypoxic lung is small, HPV will result in diversion of flow away from the hypoxic area and little or no change in pulmonary artery pressure (Fig. 7.3**A**). If, on the other hand, the hypoxic area is very large (or more so if the alveolar hypoxia is diffuse and generalized), flow cannot be diverted and the vasoconstriction results in an increased pulmonary artery pressure (Fig. 7.3**B**). Thus, for flow diversion to occur the hypoxic segment must constitute a small fraction of the total lung; i.e., flow diversion is inversely related to the size of the hypoxic segment (Fig. 7.4). The increases in pulmonary artery pressure therefore are directly related to the fraction of the total lung that is hypoxic. Thus the proportion of flow changes to pressure change decreases as the size of the hypoxic lung segment increases (Fig. 7.4). This distinction between localized and the more generalized or diffuse hypoxia is essential to understanding the nature of HPV.

The major segment of the vascular system at which HPV occurs appears to be at the level of the precapillary arterioles (30 to 50 μm).[6] These small muscular vessels are closely related to alveoli and are in an ideal position to respond

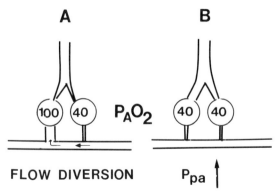

Figure 7.3. Changes in pulmonary artery pressure (Ppa) and diversion of blood flow are depicted for localized hypoxia (**A**) and for diffuse or generalized hypoxia (**B**).

to changes in alveolar oxygen concentration. Indeed, the most important stimulus to HPV appears to be the alveolar oxygen tension (P_{AO_2}). Constriction occurs as P_{AO_2} decreases below normal, and the response reaches a maximum at about 30 mm Hg. The oxygen tension in the mixed venous blood ($P_{\bar{v}O_2}$) also plays a role in the HPV response. The $P_{\bar{v}O_2}$ becomes increasingly important at very low levels of P_{AO_2} and in an atelectatic lung may be the only stimulus for HPV. At alveolar oxygen tensions above 60 mm Hg $P_{\bar{v}O_2}$ appears to have only a minor effect.[7]

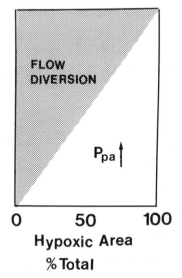

Figure 7.4. The continuity of the hypoxic pulmonary vasoconstrictive (HPV) response. With a small hypoxic segment, flow diversion away from the hypoxic segment is the principal manifestation. As the segment size increases, flow diversion decreases and the HPV response is manifested by increases in pulmonary artery pressure (Ppa). Thus, with whole-lung hypoxia the increase in Ppa is the only response.

Clinical Factors Affecting the HPV Response

A number of diverse clinical conditions diminish the HPV response (Table 7.7). Although these factors have been well identified, their mechanism of action remains unclear. Aging has been shown to produce a decrease in the magnitude of the HPV response. This inverse relationship between age and reactivity of the pulmonary vasculature exists for other pharmacologic stimuli as well.[8] Traditional consensus holds that acidosis potentiates the HPV response, while alkalosis diminishes it. However, Marshall et al.[9] have demonstrated in the isolated perfused rat lung that HPV is maximal at nearly normal pH. Although the attenuation of HPV is greater with alkalosis, the response is also reduced by acidosis, whether produced metabolically or by respiratory means.

The influence of cardiac output on HPV is such that decreases in cardiac output enhance HPV while increases attenuate the response. The increases in venous admixture associated with increased cardiac output have been ascribed to inhibition of HPV. The latter occurs because of the increase in $P\bar{v}o_2$ associated with higher cardiac outputs.

Much of the attenuation of HPV in the presence of increased intracranial pressure is attributed to the increased cardiac output and increased $P\bar{v}o_2$.[10] However, pulmonary artery pressure and left atrial pressure are increased as well. Such increased vascular pressures blunt the HPV response[11] and may explain some of the impaired gas exchange associated with other conditions, such as mitral stenosis and congestive heart failure.

Attenuation of the HPV response has been noted in many patients with chronic obstructive pulmonary disease (COPD), but the findings are quite variable.[12] The hypoxemia observed in patients with hepatic cirrhosis has also been attributed to a diminished or absent HPV response.[13] However, other reports failed to confirm these findings,[14] while still others suggest that only patients with more advanced hepatic failure exhibit reduced pulmonary vascular response to hypoxia.[15]

Table 7.7.
Clinical Conditions Associated with
Decreased HPV Response

Aging
Alkalosis
Cirrhosis
COPD
Hypothermia
Increased cardiac output
Increased intracranial pressure
Increased pulmonary artery pressure
Increased left atrial pressure
Lung inflation
Lung injury
Pneumonia

Pharmacological Modifications of HPV

Many classes of drugs alter the HPV response (Table 7.8). The β-adrenergic agonists tend to blunt HPV. Inhalation of these compounds as aerosols produces bronchodilation that is accompanied by a decreased Pao_2, presumably because of some inhibition of HPV. In contrast, α-adrenergic agonists (norepinephrine and phenylephrine) do not appear to alter HPV.

Calcium channel blockers such a nifedipine have been used as pulmonary vasodilators. Because of the resultant reduction in resting pulmonary vascular tone, the HPV response is blunted. Other vasodilator drugs have been employed to induce hypotension or reduce cardiac preload and afterload. Foremost among these are nitroprusside and nitroglycerin. Neither of these drugs appears to alter resting pulmonary artery tone, but both appear to blunt the HPV response. This attenuation of HPV has resulted in hypoxemia with nitroglycerin in normals[16] and in patients with COPD.[17]

Other vasodilators, such as minoxidil or theophylline, are also capable of inhibiting HPV. One exception among vasodilators appears to be hydralazine, which produces systemic vasodilation but does not appear to alter HPV and gas exchange.[18]

The normal HPV response appears to be augmented by compounds such as cyclooxygenase inhibitors.[19] Clinically available drugs, such as the β blocker propranolol, also appear to enhance the HPV response and improve gas exchange in acutely hypoxemic patients.[20] This apparent augmentation of HPV is associated with decreases in cardiac output and $P\bar{v}o_2$. Thus the increase in Pao_2 is largely offset by a decrease in total flow, and oxygen delivery is not actually improved.

Another drug that improves gas exchange in patients with COPD is almitrine bismesylate. The improved oxygenation occurs without significant changes in ventilation. The increase in Pao_2 is often greater than the decrease in $Paco_2$ and suggests an improved matching of ventilation and perfusion.[21] Thus it has been postulated that almitrine improves gas exchange by enhancement of HPV. Studies in normals appear to support this notion of a pharmacological enhancement of HPV by almitrine.[22]

Table 7.8.
Drug Effects on the HPV Response

Decreased HPV	Increased HPV
β-Adrenergic agonists	Almitrine bismesylate
Calcium channel blockers	Cyclooxygenase inhibitors
Inhalation anesthetics	Propranolol
Minoxidil	
Nitroglycerin	
Nitroprusside	
Theophylline	

Anesthetic Drugs and the HPV Response

Intravenous drugs of most classes used in anesthesia (opioids, barbiturates, benzodiazepines, ketamine) do not appear to have a detectable effect on the HPV response. In vitro and in vivo experiments have shown that the pulmonary vasoconstrictive response to hypoxia is maintained at blood concentrations of these drugs sufficient to produce analgesia and anesthesia.[23,24]

In vitro experiments using isolated perfused lungs have generally shown that the current halogenated inhalation agents halothane, enflurane, and isoflurane all inhibit HPV in a dose-related manner. In vitro observation with nitrous oxide suggests that it produces little or no effect on HPV.[23] Studies in intact animals, however, suggest that 70% nitrous oxide moderately diminishes the HPV response.[24,25] The halogenated anesthetics also appear to antagonize the HPV response in intact animals and humans, but widely divergent results have been reported in contrast to the in vitro experiments. The Marshalls[26] have provided a unifying concept for these findings based on the proportion of the lung that is made hypoxic. They suggest that the larger the hypoxic segment studied, the less effective will be the vasoconstriction and flow diversion away from the hypoxic site (Fig. 7.4). They have also indicated that the antagonism of HPV by inhalation anesthetics may be obscured by other hemodynamic effects.[27] The anesthetics depress myocardial function and produce a decrease in cardiac output. The latter is associated with decreased $P\overline{v}o_2$ and pulmonary artery pressures, all of which tend to intensify HPV. Thus, unless such effects are considered, the anesthetic actions on HPV may be subtle or misinterpreted.

The hypothesis that antagonism of HPV by inhalation anesthetics is important in the etiology of abnormal gas exchange during anesthesia is indeed an attractive one. However, blunting of the HPV response does not appear to sufficiently account for the impaired oxygenation observed. Inappropriately low Pao_2 values are often seen in patients breathing hyperoxic mixtures, which would be expected to provide all open alveolar units with an oxygen tension far above that at which HPV comes into play. Therefore, other factors, such as altered lung mechanics, may play a significant role in the impaired gas exchange.[27]

REFERENCES

1. Badeer HS. Gravitational effects on the distribution of pulmonary blood flow: hemodynamic misconceptions. Respiration 1982;43:408–413.
2. West JB, Dollery CT, Naimark A. Distribution of blood flow in isolated lung, relation to vascular and alveolar pressures. J Appl Physiol 1964;19:713–724.
3. Hughes JMB, Glazier JB, Maloney JE, West JB. Effect of lung volume on the distribution of pulmonary blood flow in man. Respir Physiol 1968;4:58–72.
4. Hakim TS, Dawson CA, Linehan JH. Hemodynamic response of dog lung lobe to lobar venous occlusion. J Appl Physiol 1979;47:145–152.

5. Holloway H, Perry M, Downey J, Parker J, Taylor A. Estimation of effective pulmonary capillary pressure in intact lungs. J Appl Physiol 1983;54:846–851.

6. Nagasaka Y, Bhattacharya J, Nanjo S, Gropper MA, Staub NC. Micro puncture measurements of lung microvascular pressure profile during hypoxia in cats. Circ Res 1984;54:90–95.

7. Marshall C, Marshall B. Influence of perfusate Po_2 on hypoxic pulmonary vasoconstriction in rats. Circ Res 1983;52:691–696.

8. Lowen MA, Bergman MJ, Cutaia MV, Procell RJ. Age dependent effects of chronic hypoxia on pulmonary vascular reactivity. J Appl Physiol 1987;63:1122–1129.

9. Marshall C, Lindgren L, Marshall BE. Metabolic and respiratory hydrogen ion effects on hypoxic pulmonary vasoconstriction. J Appl Physiol 1984;57:545–550.

10. Domino KB, Hlastala MP, Cheney FW. Effect of increased intracranial pressure on regional hypoxic pulmonary vasoconstriction. Anesthesiology 1990;72:490–495.

11. Benumof JL, Wahrenbrock EA. Blunted hypoxic pulmonary vasoconstriction by increased lung vascular pressures. J Appl Physiol 1975;38:846–850.

12. Weitzenblum E, Schrijen F, Mohan-Kumar T, Colas des Francs V, Lockhart A. Variability of the pulmonary vascular response to acute hypoxia in chronic bronchitis. Chest 1988;94:772–778.

13. Daoud FS, Reeves JT, Schaefer JW. Failure of hypoxic pulmonary vasoconstriction in patients with liver cirrhosis. J Clin Invest 1971;51:1076–1080.

14. Melot C, Naeije R, Dechamps P, Hallemans R, LeJeune P. Pulmonary and extrapulmonary contributors to hypoxemia in liver cirrhosis. Am Rev Respir Dis 1989;139:632–640.

15. Rodriguez-Roisin R, Roca J, Agusti AG, Mastai R, Wagner P, Bosch J. Gas exchange and pulmonary vascular reactivity patients with liver cirrhosis. Am Rev Respir Dis 1987;135:1085–1092.

16. Hales CA, Westphal D. Hypoxemia following the administration of sublingual nitroglycerin. Am J Med 1978;65:911–918.

17. Chick TW, Kochukoshy KN, Matsumoto S, Leach JK. The effect of nitroglycerin on gas exchange, hemodynamics and oxygen transport in patients with chronic obstructive pulmonary disease. Am J Med Sci 1978;276:105–111.

18. Ghignone M, Girling L, Prewitt RM. Effects of hydralazine on cardiopulmonary function in canine low pressure pulmonary edema. Anesthesiology 1983;59:187–190.

19. Leeman M, Naeije R, LeJeune P, Melot C. Influence of cyclooxygenase inhibition and of leukotriene receptor blockade on pulmonary vascular pressure: cardiac index relationships in hyperoxic and hypoxic dogs. Clin Sci (Lond) 1987;72:717–724.

20. Vincent JL, Lignian J, Gillet JB, Berre J, Contu E. Increase in Pao_2 following intravenous administration of propranolol in acutely hypoxemic patients. Chest 1985;88:558–562.

21. Melot C, Naeije R, Rothschold T, Mertens T, Mols P, Halleman R. Improvement in ventilation perfusion matching by almitrine in chronic obstructive pulmonary disease. Chest 1983;83:528–533.

22. Melot C, Dechamps P, Hallemans R, Decroly P, Mols P. Enhancement of hypoxic pulmonary vasoconstriction by low dose almitrine bismesylate in normal humans. Am Rev Respir Dis 1989;139:111–119.

23. Bjertaines LJ. Hypoxia-induced vasoconstriction in isolated perfused lungs exposed to injectable or intravenous anesthetics. Acta Anaesthesiol Scand 1977;21:133–147.

24. Benumof JL, Wahrenbrock EA. Local effects of anesthetics on regional hypoxic pulmonary vasoconstriction. Anesthesiology 1975;43:525–532.

25. Mathers J, Benumof JL, Wahrenbrock EA. General anesthetics and regional hypoxic pulmonary vasoconstriction. Anesthesiology 1977;46:111–114.

26. Marshall BE, Marshall C. Continuity of response to hypoxic pulmonary vasoconstriction. J Appl Physiol 1980;49:189–196.

27. Marshall BE, Marshall C. Anesthesia and the pulmonary circulation. In: Covino BG, Fozzard HA, Rehder K, Stricharz GR, eds. Effects of anesthesia. Bethesda MD: American Physiological Society, 1985:121–136.

Chapter 8

Respiratory Gas Exchange

Overall gas exchange is reflected by the composition of the arterial blood. The gas content of arterial blood represents a weighted average of all the gas-exchanging units in the lungs. Thus, the blood leaving each alveolus has an oxygen and carbon dioxide tension that reflects the composition of the alveolar gas and the efficiency with which the incoming pulmonary blood flow is able to equilibrate. Anesthetic drugs and techniques can significantly alter this process, and the effects are often compounded by preexisting disease and other acute events. This chapter provides insight into the nature and mechanism of these gas exchange abnormalities and examines some of their consequences.

CARBON DIOXIDE ELIMINATION

Fundamental Determinants of CO_2 Tensions

The carbon dioxide that is removed by alveolar ventilation is constantly added to the alveolar gas from the pulmonary circulation. The CO_2 tension in the arterial blood (Pa_{O_2}) is the net result of the balance between the metabolic rate of O_2 production by body tissues ($\dot{V}_{CO_2}$) and the rate at which the lungs excrete CO_2 via alveolar ventilation ($\dot{V}_A$). The Pa_{CO_2} is directly proportional to $\dot{V}_{CO_2}$ and inversely proportional to $\dot{V}_A$. This relationship can be expressed as:

$$Pa_{CO_2} = K \cdot \frac{\dot{V}_{CO_2}}{\dot{V}_A}$$

The proportionality constant (K) is equal to 0.863 when $\dot{V}_{CO_2}$ is expressed in milliliters per minute as a dry gas at standard temperature and pressure (STPD) and $\dot{V}_A$ is expressed in liters per minute as a saturated gas at body temperature and pressure (BTPS). The K value allows the simultaneous conversion of concentration to partial pressure and corrects for units that conventionally express the gas volumes.

124

This equation simply states that under the ideal conditions of a steady state the CO_2 output is matched by the alveolar ventilation. If $\dot{V}A$ is depressed for some reason, $Paco_2$ must rise in proportion to this decreased $\dot{V}A$. This inverse relationship between $\dot{V}A$ and $Paco_2$ is described by a rectangular hyperbola (see Fig. 4.1). In many clinical settings, however, this simple relationship is modified by other factors that result in an increase in $Paco_2$ above normal (>46 mm Hg) to produce hypercapnia.

Hypercapnia with Normal Lung Function

Endogenous CO_2 production may increase with such conditions as fever, sepsis, seizures, hyperthyroidism, or total parenteral nutrition with a very high glucose intake.[1] Unless ventilation is increased accordingly, CO_2 elevations may occur in such patients.

Occasionally, nonmetabolic sources for CO_2 may be present. For example, an increase in $Paco_2$ may be observed following CO_2 instillation for laparoscopy. Similarly, transient elevations in $Paco_2$ occur after the administration of sodium bicarbonate if ventilation is not allowed to increase.[2] More common and perhaps more dangerous is an increased CO_2 in the inspired gas. Whether this results from anesthetic mishaps such as failure of soda lime absorber, incompetent valves in the circle system, or merely breathing in confined spaces, a new steady state will be achieved. This new level of $Paco_2$ will be defined by the quantity of CO_2 in the inspired air, the CO_2 generated by metabolism, and the relative change in alveolar ventilation.

How the system responds to increased alveolar ventilation is a crucial determinant of how adequately CO_2 is eliminated. Alveolar hypoventilation may result in hypercapnia whether or not respiratory system disease is present. The responsiveness of the respiratory control system to CO_2 is an important determinant of $Paco_2$. This respiratory controller is affected by a wide variety of disease states and drugs. These are discussed in more detail elsewhere (see Chapters 4 to 6). Signals arising in the respiratory controller must produce a response in the respiratory system bellows. If the respiratory muscles are weak or easily fatigued, the respiratory drive will not be translated in adequate levels of ventilation. Similarly, if the muscles must overcome an increased mechanical workload because of decreased compliance or increased resistance of the respiratory system, CO_2 retention may occur also.

Hypercapnia with Impaired Lung Function

Retention of carbon dioxide occurs more commonly when there is disturbance of the gas exchange function of the lung. Net effective alveolar ventilation can be decreased even if total ventilation is increased. This situation results either because significant portions of the lung are not perfused and function as a "dead space" or disease is severe enough to significantly affect the matching of ventilation and perfusion.

The alveolar ventilation, which influences the level of Pa_{CO_2}, cannot be measured directly but must be derived from another volume, the minute volume ($\dot{V}E$). The alveolar ventilation differs from this volume of air that moves in and out of the lungs each minute by an amount of gas that does not participate in the exchange of CO_2 with the blood. This volume of gas is usually referred to as the physiologic dead space. However, some have preferred to term this "wasted ventilation," since this portion of each breath is literally wasted with respect to its contribution to gas exchange.

A portion of this dead space gas is contained within the conducting airways from the mouth and nose down to the terminal bronchioles and is termed the anatomic dead space. In a normal adult this consists of about one-third of the volume of each breath. The anatomic dead space (V_D) is larger in males than females, presumably because of body size and lung volume. The anatomic V_D is larger in older men than younger men because of the increase in end-expiratory lung volume (FRC) seen with advancing age. In general, anatomic V_D is affected by changes in airway caliber and increases with increasing lung volume. The average increase appears to be 2 to 3 ml per 100 ml increase in lung volume.[3] Other factors that influence the size of the upper airway affect V_D. These include positioning of the neck and jaw and the presence of artificial oral airways. Finally, tracheal intubation, which decreases the volume of the upper airway, and tracheostomy, which bypasses the upper airway, also serve to decrease anatomic V_D.

The other portion of the physiologic dead space, the alveolar dead space, may be defined as the part of the inspired gas that passes through the conducting airways to mix with gas at the alveolar level but does not actively participate in gas exchange. The alveolar dead space results from a lack of effective perfusion of the airspaces to which inspired gas is distributed. Factors such as reduced cardiac output, hypovolemia, hypotension, and pulmonary embolism tend to reduce pulmonary blood flow. Thus they increase the alveolar dead space fraction and impair CO_2 excretion.

The sum of the combined anatomic and alveolar components, the physiologic dead space, cannot be measured directly but can be calculated from CO_2 tensions in simultaneously collected samples of mixed expired air ($P\bar{E}_{CO_2}$) and arterial blood (Pa_{CO_2}). The formula used to calculate the fraction of wasted ventilation per breath or, more specifically, the ratio of physiologic dead space (V_D) to tidal volume (V_T) is a modification of the classic Bohr equation proposed by Enghoff. In this equation alveolar CO_2 tension (PA_{CO_2}) is replaced by Pa_{CO_2}. The expired gas is a mixture of dead space gas and that from the gas-exchanging compartment. Since dead space gas contains essentially no CO_2 the quantity of CO_2 expired should come entirely from the gas-exchanging compartment.

$$V_T \times P\bar{E}_{CO_2} \quad = \quad (V_T - V_D) \times Pa_{CO_2}$$

| Amount of CO_2 expired | Amount expired from gas-exchanging compartment |

By solving for V_D/V_T, this can be expressed as:

$$\frac{V_D}{V_T} = \frac{Pa_{CO_2} - P\bar{E}_{CO_2}}{Pa_{CO_2}}$$

Typical values for V_D/V_T in healthy subjects are about 0.30, so nearly one-third of the inspired V_T does not participate in gas exchange. In diseased lungs V_D/V_T increases and values greater than 0.75 may be observed.

The concept of dead space (V_D) and ventilation-perfusion ($\dot{V}_A/\dot{Q}$) mismatch involve a continuum in which V_D implies the most extreme mismatch in which the $\dot{V}_A/\dot{Q}$ ratio reaches infinity. If such a large increase in ventilation-perfusion mismatch cannot be compensated for by increasing ventilation, Pa_{CO_2} will of necessity rise. A less common malfunction of CO_2 excretion results when large areas of right-to-left shunt or low $\dot{V}_A/\dot{Q}$ are present. Here the CO_2 in mixed venous blood enters the arterial system without the opportunity for excretion via a ventilated alveolus. Again ventilation must increase to compensate for this inefficiency in CO_2 excretion.

In patients with chronic obstructive pulmonary disease, hypercapnia appears to be more the result of this ventilation-perfusion mismatch than the result of actual decreases in ventilation.[4] Such patients who remain normocapneic must compensate for this mismatch by increasing total minute ventilation to very high levels. Such increased levels of ventilation may achieve normocapnia but invariably do so at the expense of an excessively increased work of breathing in the presence of airflow obstruction.

Physiologic Consequences of Hypercapnia

There are no specific clinical diagnostic signs of hypercapnia. The varied signs and symptoms include headache, nausea, sweating, flushing, restlessness, tachypnea, and, with marked hypercapnia (>90 mm Hg), unconsciousness. These reflect the actions of CO_2 on the respiratory, cardiovascular, and central nervous system functions.

Respiratory Effects. As Pa_{CO_2} rises to produce hypercapnia, CO_2 excretion is less than its production. As a steady state arises, excretion must equal production. Thus the ventilatory response to CO_2 (increased $\dot{V}_E$) must take place or Pa_{CO_2} will continue to rise further until severe hypercapnia ($Pa_{CO_2} > 90$) ensues and depresses respiration. The ventilatory response to CO_2 characteristic in the awake patient is blunted, though not completely eliminated, during general anesthesia (see Chapter 6).

Hypercapnia may affect respiratory gas exchange by its mild effect on pulmonary vasoconstriction[5] or by depression of diaphragmatic function.[6] In addition, the reduced alveolar ventilation associated with increased Pa_{CO_2} may also be inadequate to deliver oxygen to the alveoli to replace that taken off by the pulmonary blood flow. Thus the oxygen tension in the alveoli (PA_{O_2}) decreases and in turn produces a reduction in Pa_{O_2}. This secondary effect of hypercapnia is also associated with a shift of the oxyhemoglobin dissociation curve to the right. The rightward shift further decreases oxygen saturation at any given level of Pao_2. However, this decreased affinity of hemoglobin for oxygen does facilitate unloading of oxygen from blood to tissues at a higher Pao_2.

Cardiovascular Effects.   Many of the circulatory effects of hypercapnia appear to enhance oxygen delivery and CO_2 removal at the tissue level. The direct effect of CO_2 and the accompanying acidosis on the heart and blood vessels is to depress the function of smooth and cardiac muscle. The result is decreased cardiac contractility and, in most vascular beds, vasodilation. The one exception of course is the pulmonary circulation, which tends to constrict.

In healthy individuals the direct effects of CO_2 are modified by those of central sympathetic stimulation, which result in tachycardia, mild hypertension, and increased myocardial contractility. With disease states that depress autonomic responsiveness, and with most anesthetics, much of this sympathetic stimulation is obtunded and the direct depressant effects of acidosis on the tissues are manifested.

Central Nervous System Effects.   Hypercapnia affects central nervous system function by its stimulating effect on breathing. The excess CO_2 also acts on the cerebral vascular bed to produce vasodilation. In the presence of cerebral pathology the vasodilation within the closed cranial space may produce dangerous increases in intracranial pressure. Higher CO_2 tensions depress general neuronal activity and produce a state of unconsciousness not unlike that of general anesthesia.

Physiological Consequences of Hypocapnia

Alveolar hyperventilation from any cause will result in decreased CO_2 tension (hypocapnia). This hypocapnia may decrease cardiac output by decreasing sympathetic activity, ionized calcium, or coronary blood flow. At the same time a leftward shift of the oxyhemoglobin dissociation curve (increased affinity for O_2) will result in reduced ability to give up O_2 at the tissue level. This necessitates an increased cardiac output to maintain the same rate of O_2 delivery. Vasoconstriction of cerebral and spinal cord vessels may also have undesirable effects. To add to this, hypocapnia may further increase oxygen consumption in the face of a decreased tissue oxygen supply.

Hypocapnia also decreases ionized calcium and serum potassium concentrations. The latter, for example, changes by about 1.5 mEq/liter with each 10 mm Hg change in $Paco_2$ as a result of altered potassium distribution between intracellular and extracellular spaces.[7]

Further abnormalities in gas exchange may occur in response to reduction in CO_2 tension. Disturbances in ventilation-perfusion matching may develop if hypocapnia inhibits hypoxic pulmonary vasoconstriction. Local increases in airway resistance may also occur in normals and patients with lung disease.[8] This bronchoconstriction appears to be a response to the reduction in alveolar

CO_2 tension, which in a sense is analogous to the vascular response to reduced alveolar O_2 tension.

Some of the physiological impact of hypocapnia relates to the difference in time course associated with acute hyperventilation as opposed to hypoventilation. The $Paco_2$ tends to decrease far more rapidly during hyperventilation than a similar increase occurs in $Paco_2$ during hypoventilation. Following hyperventilation 50% of the decrease in $Paco_2$ occurs in about 3 minutes, while a 50% increase in $Paco_2$ takes nearly 20 minutes following a decrease in ventilation.[9] During complete apnea $Paco_2$ rises 8 to 15 mm Hg in the first minute or so and exhibits a subsequent linear increase of about 3 mm Hg/min.[10]

OXYGENATION

Whenever the supply of oxygen to the tissues is unable to meet metabolic demands, hypoxia results. Hypoxia has been variously subdivided into hypoxic, stagnant, anemic, and histotoxic types. Stagnant hypoxia is produced when blood flow to the tissues is reduced, whereas anemic hypoxia results from a decreased oxygen-carrying capacity because of low hemoglobin or binding of hemoglobin with other substances (e.g., carbon monoxide). If the cell is unable to use oxygen to produce energy, the term histotoxic hypoxia is applied. Such hypoxia can result from cyanide toxicity and, unlike the other forms of hypoxia, is characterized by an increase in mixed venous oxygen tension since tissues cannot utilize the oxygen presented to them.

By far the most common variant of hypoxia encountered clinically is hypoxic hypoxia. This is associated with an abnormally low arterial oxygen tension (Pao_2), which is referred to as hypoxemia. The causes of hypoxemia are many and varied and must take into account factors such as inspired O_2 concentration, alveolar CO_2 tension, barometric pressure, patient age, and the presence of lung disease.

Alveolar Gas Composition

The alveolar gas content is influenced by the matching of ventilation and blood flow and by the composition of the mixed venous blood. First and foremost, however, the composition of gas in the alveoli depends on the content of the gas that is inspired. The partial pressure of each gas in this inspired mixture is proportional to the fractional concentration of the gas. As gases enter the respiratory tract they are warmed to body temperature and humidified. Thus, it is necessary to take into account the partial pressure exerted by water vapor (P_{H_2O}) at body temperature, which is usually 47 mm Hg. Thus the fractional concentration of oxygen in the inspired air (Fio_2), which is expressed as a dry gas, can be used to calculate the inspired oxygen tension (Pio_2) within the trachea:

$$Pio_2 = Fio_2 (PB - 47) \text{ mm Hg}$$

For clinical purposes it is sufficient to use the standard barometric pressure (P_B) at sea level, 760 mm Hg, to calculate P_{IO_2}. Thus in a subject breathing room air,

$$P_{IO_2} = 0.21 \ (760 - 47) = 150 \ \text{mm Hg}$$

The differences in gas composition between ambient air and that in the trachea are listed in Table 8.1. The total pressure of gas in the trachea and alveoli is equal to the atmospheric pressure (Table 8.1). Since there is no exchange of nitrogen within the respiratory tract, the partial pressure of nitrogen is the same in the alveoli and the trachea. The oxygen tension in the alveoli (P_{AO_2}), however, will be less than the P_{IO_2} in the trachea because CO_2 is added to the alveoli from mixed venous blood. The P_{AO_2} therefore will differ from the P_{IO_2} by an amount directly related to the quantity of CO_2 added. If the CO_2 volume added by the blood equals the oxygen taken up by the blood, than P_{AO_2} may be calculated simply as follows:

$$P_{AO_2} = P_{IO_2} - P_{ACO_2}$$

Usually the ratio of CO_2 produced to the O_2 consumed, the respiratory exchange ratio (R), is less than 1.0. If one assumes that R approximates 0.8 and also assumes that ideal P_{ACO_2} can be estimated by arterial CO_2 tension (P_{aCO_2}), the alveolar gas equation can be simplified for clinical uses as:

$$P_{AO_2} = P_{IO_2} = P_{aCO_2}/0.8$$

CAUSES OF HYPOXEMIA

Normal Lung Function.   When there is no impairment of lung function, hypoxemia may result from a variety of factors, which include low inspired O_2

Table 8.1.
Approximate Partial Pressure (mm Hg) for Respiratory Tract Gases in a Young Healthy Adult Breathing Room Air ($F_{IO_2} = 0.2$)

Gas	Ambient Air	Trachea	Alveoli
O_2	150	150	100
CO_2	0	0	40
H_2O	20[a]	47	47
N_2	590	563	573
Total	760	760	760

[a]Water vapor pressure varies with humidity and exacts a proportionate change in the partial pressures of oxygen (P_{O_2}) and nitrogen (P_{N_2}).

concentration (FIO_2), hypoventilation, decreased cardiac output, a shift in the O_2 hemoglobin dissociation curve, and decreased hemoglobin concentration. By far the most dangerous but easily correctable cause of hypoxemia is a low FIO_2. Any decreases in inspired O_2 concentration below that of normal ambient air will result in hypoxemia. The alveolar oxygen tension will be increased or decreased by an amount determined by the Po_2 of the inspired gas if other factors remain constant. The alveolar to arterial O_2 difference ($AaDo_2$), however, will not be increased.

The PAO_2 can also be decreased by a diminished alveolar ventilation, whether due to airway obstruction or drug-induced depression of breathing. The simplified alveolar air equation suggests that as CO_2 tension increases, PAO_2 will decrease by a similar amount. Thus, unless FIO_2 is increased above 0.21 hypoxemia can result from hypoventilation. Again, as in the case of decreased FIO_2, the $AaDo_2$ will not be increased.

The effect of increasing FIO_2 from 0.21 to 0.30 is shown in Figure 8.1. The improvement in PAO_2 at any level of ventilation of $PACO_2$ is about 64 mm Hg. Thus at the high levels of $PACO_2$ associated with marked hypoventilation, an FIO_2 of 0.30 appears to be the maximum O_2 concentration required to correct the hypoxemia present with the ambient air.

The PAO_2 can be influenced by a decrease in cardiac output, which in the absence of other changes may temporarily increase PAO_2 because less blood flows through the lungs to remove O_2 from the alveolar gas. More importantly, the reduced cardiac output is associated with increased tissue O_2 extraction, which results in a reduced O_2 content in the mixed venous blood. As the blood passes through the lungs with its reduced O_2 content the resultant Pao_2 is decreased compared to that with a normal cardiac output. Abnormal O_2 trans-

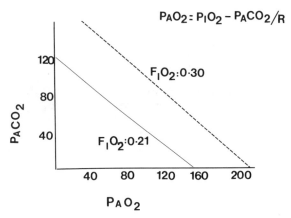

Figure 8.1. O_2-CO_2 diagram based on the simplified alveolar air equation for ambient air (FIO_2 = 0.21) at sea level (atmospheric pressure = 760 mm Hg) is indicated by the *solid line*, while that for an enriched O_2 mixture (FIO_2 = 0.30) is indicated by the *dotted line*. An R value of 0.8 was used to calculate both lines.

port, because of decreased hemoglobin concentration or rightward shifts of the oxyhemoglobin dissociation curve, can also lead to increased O_2 extraction by tissues and a similar reduction in mixed venous and arterial oxygen tensions.

Abnormal Lung Function.   When hypoxemia occurs in the presence of a normal or increased P_{AO_2}, it can only result from disturbances in the normal gas exchange function of the lung. This interference with the lung's ability to oxygenate blood consists of three basic abnormalities:

1. *Diffusion*—an impaired movement of gas (O_2) from alveolus to capillary.
2. *Shunt*—the presence of channels (extrapulmonary and pulmonary) that allow venous blood to bypass the normal gas exchange units in the lung.
3. *Ventilation-perfusion mismatch*—poor matching of blood and gas at the alveolar level.

Diffusion Abnormality.   Normally O_2 and CO_2 equilibrate between blood and gas phases in far less time than it takes the red cell to traverse the pulmonary capillary network. Thus diffusion limitation plays a very small role in normal gas exchange at rest unless F_{IO_2} is reduced, such as at high altitude. During vigorous exercise, however, some patients can develop a decreased P_{AO_2} because the increased velocity of blood flow through the pulmonary capillaries shortens the time available for diffusion equilibrium. While this abnormal diffusion can be caused by thickening of the air-blood interface (alveolar-capillary block), it more commonly results from a reduction in pulmonary capillary blood volume. The latter state differs from the thickened membrane in that as capillaries are destroyed or obstructed, others are recruited and the flow velocity through these remaining vessels increases. Thus, with severe disease (e.g., emphysema) the time available for gas exchange at rest may be as short as with exercise, and equilibration of gas fails to occur adequately. This of course can be offset easily by increasing the driving pressure for O_2 (i.e., the P_{AO_2}) by using oxygen-enriched mixtures.

Shunts.   Another interference with ideal gas exchange occurs in the form of right-to-left shunts. Normally a small amount of venous blood bypasses the right ventricle and empties directly into the left atrium. This "anatomic shunt" represents venous return from pleural, bronchial, and thebesian veins, which constitutes as much as 5% of total cardiac output. Right-to-left shunts of greater magnitude occur with cyanotic congenital heart disease.

In addition to these discrete anatomic pathways, a shunt effect may be produced by normal vessels that perfuse areas of lung that are not ventilated because the airways are closed or the conducting airways are obstructed. The term "shunt effect" or "venous admixture" is generally applied to these lung units whose ventilation is maximally decreased compared to the amount of perfusion. The venous admixture is manifested clinically by hypoxemia that is responsive to increased inspired O_2 concentrations. In diseases associated with major areas of lung without ventilation (absolute shunt) or in the case of the anatomic shunts the hypoxemia is refractory to O_2 administration.

Ventilation-Perfusion Imbalance.   The distribution of ventilation and pulmonary blood flow is neither uniform nor proportionate even in normal lungs. This nonuniform distribution of ventilation and perfusion results in impaired gas exchange. The primary effect of ventilation-perfusion mismatch is an impairment of oxygenation. The high Pao_2 of lung regions with high ventilation-perfusion ratios are able to produce only a minimal increase in the O_2 content of the blood because of the relatively flat oxyhemoglobin dissociation curve in that range of partial pressure (Fig. 8.2). Hence these areas are unable to compensate for regions with low $\dot{V}A/\dot{Q}$ values. CO_2 elimination is also impaired by ventilation-perfusion mismatching, but the elevated CO_2 stimulates ventilation. Because the CO_2 dissociation curve is nearly linear in the physiologic range, this increased ventilation is able to compensate for low ventilation-perfusion areas and maintain CO_2 near normal. With severe ventilation-perfusion mismatch or impaired ability to increase ventilation, this compensation is inadequate to avoid an increase in CO_2.

Physiologic Consequences of Hypoxemia

Foremost among the clinical manifestations of hypoxemia is cyanosis, which marks the presence of a significant amount of desaturated hemoglobin (usually > 5 g/100 ml). Although it is rather subjective, cyanosis is usually observed with hemoglobin saturations less than 85%. This is usually associated with a

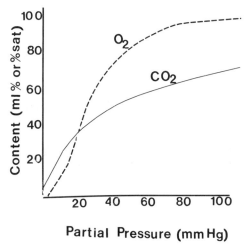

Figure 8.2.   The sigmoid shape of the O_2 dissociation curve *(dashed line)* is contrasted with that of the relatively linear CO_2 dissociation curve *(solid line)* to illustrate how hyperventilation is able to lower CO_2 tension and content almost in linear fashion. In contrast, increasing O_2 tension has little effect on increasing O_2 content in the normal range because of the sigmoid shape of the curve.

Pao_2 of 45 to 50 mm Hg in the adult, while in the infant because of the leftward shift of the oxyhemoglobin dissociation curve it may correspond to a Pao_2 of 35 to 40 mm Hg. Cyanosis may be apparent without actual hypoxemia, as in methemoglobinemia and sulfhemoglobinemia, and conversely may not be apparent in the presence of anemia or intense peripheral vasoconstriction. Thus the diagnosis of hypoxemia is established with certainty only when O_2 saturation or Pao_2 is measured.

Hypoxemia is associated with an increased minute ventilation, largely through an increased respiratory rate. This brisk response to a low Pao_2 resides in the carotid bodies and is very sensitive to the depressive effects of the volatile anesthetics (see Chapter 6). These anesthetics exert a similar blunting effect on the circulatory responses to hypoxia. The latter responses also appear to be mediated via the carotid bodies. The circulatory compensation to hypoxia acts to redistribute blood flow and maintain arterial pressure. The aim is to increase the quantity of O_2 carried to important tissues and consists largely of an increased heart rate and cardiac output with vasodilation in the brain and heart, while the muscle beds and splanchnic circulation undergo constriction.

Ultimately, the consequences of hypoxia manifest themselves by a disruption of the function of all major organ systems. The cerebral cortex, which begins to cease functioning after about 30 seconds of hypoxia, may suffer irreversible damage after 5 minutes. The heart takes about 5 minutes to cease functioning and experiences tissue death after about 10 minutes.

INDICES OF THE EFFICIENCY OF OXYGENATION

Rational interpretation and treatment of reduced Pao_2 values requires some estimation of the oxygenating capacity of the lungs. The calculation of venous admixtures or physiologic shunt ($\dot{Q}s/\dot{Q}t$) has been used to express the portion of the cardiac output that perfuses regions that do not participate in delivering oxygen to the blood. To calculate this shunt, one must know barometric pressure, Pao_2, $Paco_2$, hemoglobin (Hb) concentration, and mixed venous O_2 tension ($P\bar{v}o_2$). Thus equipment must consist of a blood gas analyzer, blood sampling devices, and either a pulmonary artery or central venous catheter to obtain $P\bar{v}o_2$. To calculate true shunt it is also necessary to ensure that the patient is breathing 100% O_2 for at least 20 minutes.

The formula used to calculate shunt is:

$$\dot{Q}s/\dot{Q}t = \frac{C\bar{c}o_2 - Cao_2}{C\bar{c}o_2 - C\bar{v}o_2}$$

where $C\bar{c}o_2$ is the O_2 content of ventilated and perfused pulmonary capillaries; Cao_2, is the O_2 content of arterial blood; and $C\bar{v}o_2$ is the O_2 content of mixed venous blood.

Since perfused capillaries ventilated with O_2 are exposed to the P_{AO_2}, the latter must be calculated from the alveolar air equation. The P_{AO_2} is multiplied by the solubility coefficient (0.003) to calculate dissolved O_2. Since each gram of hemoglobin also holds 1.39 ml of O_2 when fully saturated, $C\overline{c}_{O_2} = (Hb \times 1.39) + (P_{AO_2} \times 0.003)$.

Arterial Hb is not fully saturated, therefore $Ca_{O_2} = (Hb \times 1.39 \times \%sat) + (Pa_{O_2} \times 0.003)$.

Mixed venous O_2 content is calculated in similar fashion in that $P\overline{v}_{O_2}$ is multiplied by 0.003 to estimate dissolved O_2. Thus, $C\overline{v}_{O_2} = (Hb \times 1.39 \times \%sat) + (P\overline{v}_{O_2} \times 0.003)$.

The accuracy of $\dot{Q}s/\dot{Q}t$ calculations depend on many variables, such as cardiac output, respiratory quotient, the quality of the mixed venous sample, or an assumed arterial venous O_2 content difference. Like other indices of oxygenation, $\dot{Q}s/\dot{Q}t$ is also influenced by ventilation-perfusion mismatch, F_{IO_2}, and variations in mixed venous O_2 content. If alveoli are actually ventilated the calculated shunt should approach the normal value of about 5%, since the F_{IO_2} of 1.00 minimizes the effects of ventilation-perfusion mismatch. Thus, abnormally high $\dot{Q}s/\dot{Q}t$ values are due primarily to blood flow through completely unventilated areas in the lung.

When pulmonary artery catheters are not in use several simplified measures have been used at the bedside to assess the efficiency of oxygenation. The alveolar to arterial O_2 tension difference (AaD_{O_2}) has been used extensively as an index of gas exchange, largely because it is easy to estimate. Some clinicians have used AaD_{O_2} in a shortcut method for calculating shunt assuming unchanged cardiac output and an F_{IO_2} or 1.00.[11]

$$\% \text{ shunt} = \frac{AaD_{O_2}}{10}$$

This simplified relationship does not appear to be valid, however, since the relationship between $\dot{Q}s/\dot{Q}t\%$ and AaD_{O_2} is not linear over the range of clinically important shunts (10 to 50%).[12]

The AaD_{O_2} is less than 10 mm Hg in normal young persons breathing ambient air. This increases linearly to about 25 mm Hg in the 70- to 80-year-old. More importantly, AaD_{O_2} increases as F_{IO_2} is increased, both in normals[13] and in patients with pulmonary disease.[14] This variability with changes in F_{IO_2} limits the usefulness for comparing gas exchange in patients receiving a different level of F_{IO_2} and interpreting changes in a single patient as F_{IO_2} is increased or decreased.

One attempt to standardize Pa_{O_2} values obtained with a different F_{IO_2} has been to use the ratio of Pa_{O_2} to F_{IO_2} (P/F). This is easily calculated, but the units are confusing. F_{IO_2} values less than 1.0 result in a P/F ratio that is expressed in mm Hg but has a higher value than the Pa_{O_2}. The P/F value also does not take into account the effect of different levels of Pa_{CO_2}.

Another simply calculated index of oxygenation is the ratio of arterial to alveolar O_2 tensions (a/APo_2). This does account for changes in $Paco_2$ due to ventilation and appears to be equal to $1 - (AaDo_2/PAo_2)$.[15] Thus it resembles the P/F ratio in correcting for changes in Fio_2. The two ratios are also similar in that they are useful bedside indices that do not require central sampling for mixed venous blood. Both, however, tend to lose their reliability as the percent of shunt increases.[16]

Another calculated value purported to improve the accuracy of $AaDo_2$[17] to estimate $\dot{V}A/\dot{Q}$ abnormalities is the "respiratory index."[17] This is derived by dividing the $AaDo_2$ by Pao_2. While some have considered the respiratory index clinically useful,[18] other data strongly suggest that it is not the variable of choice for assessing the adequacy of oxygenation.[16]

ANALYSIS OF VENTILATION-PERFUSION DISTRIBUTIONS

The gas exchange in each alveolus is determined by the relationships between ventilation $(\dot{V}A)$ and perfusion $(\dot{Q})$. These relationships have been characterized in a lung model consisting of three basic compartments. The lowest possible $\dot{V}A/\dot{Q}$ ratio (i.e., zero) is represented by the shunt compartment consisting of unventilated but perfused alveoli. The largest $\dot{V}A/\dot{Q}$ ratios (i.e., infinity) are represented by dead space, which represents alveoli that are ventilated but essentially not perfused. The third compartment represents the continuum of relationships between $\dot{V}A$ and $\dot{Q}$.

The shunt and dead space compartments can be estimated from calculations previously described in this chapter. Efforts to characterize the continuous distribution of $\dot{V}A/\dot{Q}$ reached fruition with the multiple inert gas elimination technique developed by Wagner et al.[19] In this technique six inert gases (i.e., gases that do not combine with hemoglobin) are dissolved in saline or dextrose for intravenous administration. These six gases, in order of increasing solubility in the blood, are sulfur hexafluoride, ethane, cyclopropane, halothane, diethyl ether, and acetone. The principle of the technique is based on the assumption that if such gases are delivered to a lung unit from the mixed venous blood, the relative retention of such gases by blood passing through an alveolus depends on the solubility or blood-gas partition coefficient (λ) and the $\dot{V}A/\dot{Q}$ ratio. The fractional retention (R) of a gas, which is the ratio between arterial tension (Pa) and mixed venous tension $(P\bar{v})$ can be expressed by the following equation:

$$R = \frac{\lambda}{\lambda + \dot{V}A/\dot{Q}}$$

A similar equation can be generated for the excretion (E) of a gas, which is the relationship between alveolar tension (PA) and mixed venous tension $(P\bar{v})$.

It is evident from the equation that when the λ for a given gas equals the $\dot{V}_A/\dot{Q}$ of the alveolus, the retention will be equal to 0.5, i.e., half of the gas will be retained and half eliminated. If a gas with a higher λ enters the same $\dot{V}_A/\dot{Q}$ lung unit, more of that gas will be retained while a gas with a lower λ will be retained less. Similarly, an increase in $\dot{V}_A$ or decrease in $\dot{Q}$ (i.e., increased $\dot{V}_A/\dot{Q}$) will also result in decreased retention of the gas. Increased retention or decreased excretion of the gas may result from a decreased $\dot{V}_A$ or increased $\dot{Q}$ (i.e., decreased $\dot{V}_A/\dot{Q}$).

Graphs can be constructed for the retention (Pa/P$\bar{v}$) and excretion of PA/Pv) as a function of the solubility of a gas (blood-gas partition coefficient). Such plots (Fig. 8.3) provide information about the distribution of $\dot{V}_A/\dot{Q}$ ratios in the lung. If lung contains areas perfused but not ventilated (shunt), the retention of the least soluble gases is increased (Fig. 8.3**A**). On the other hand, in the presence of very high $\dot{V}_A/\dot{Q}$ ratios the gases of very high solubility will be affected; their excretion is decreased (Fig. 8.3**B**).

The retention and excretion data for the inert gases must be transformed into $\dot{V}_A/\dot{Q}$ distributions. The problems and limitations of this transformation are a subject of much controversy and are well beyond the scope of this presentation. The reader should refer to the original publications[19] and subsequent arguments,[20] as well as a concise review.[21] It will become quite evident that, despite its limitations, the multiple inert gas elimination technique represents a valuable conceptual tool to analyze pulmonary gas exchange.

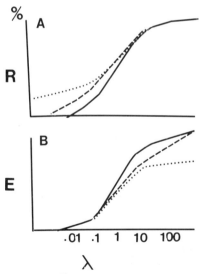

Figure 8.3. Retention (R) (i.e., arterial/mixed venous) and excretion (E) (i.e., alveolar/mixed venous) curves as a function of solubility expressed as blood gas partition coefficient (λ) are plotted for homogeneous lung *(solid lines)* and with low $\dot{V}_A/\dot{Q}$ areas *(dashed line)* and shunt *(dotted line)* are shown in *A*, while those with high $\dot{V}_A/\dot{Q}$ areas *(dashed line)* and dead space *(dotted line)* are shown in *B*.

IMPAIRED GAS EXCHANGE DURING GENERAL ANESTHESIA

The abnormal pulmonary gas exchange associated with general anesthesia is manifested by an increased alveolar-arterial O_2 tension gradient. The impaired oxygenation and to some extent the CO_2 elimination appear to be a reflection of an increased ventilation-perfusion mismatch, right-to-left intrapulmonary shunting, and an increase in alveolar dead space. All of these changes tend to be increased substantially in the presence of preexisting lung disease.[22] A number of theories have been proposed to account for these changes, many based on the changes in respiratory mechanics associated with general anesthesia. Foremost among these are the reduction in functional residual capacity and alterations in the distribution of ventilation.

Reduction in Functional Residual Capacity

In supine subjects the induction of general anesthesia reduces FRC such that end-expiratory volume decreases close to residual volume. This FRC may lie below the closing capacity, i.e., the volume associated with dependent airway closure or, more precisely, dynamic flow limitation.[23] Early observations with halothane anesthesia suggested a correlation between the degree of impaired oxygenation and the reduction in FRC[24] and led to the hypothesis that airway closure and atelectasis were the consequences of a reduced FRC.

One important aspect of the theory of airway closure lies in the assumption that closing capacity (CC) remains the same in both the anesthetized and awake states. The decrease in lung compliance in the anesthetized state reflects an increased elastic recoil. Airway closure to a great extent is due to a decrease in lung elastic recoil. As a result, one might expect a decrease in closing capacity with general anesthesia. Initial reports suggested no difference in closing capacity between awake and anesthetized states.[25,26] Subsequent work, however, provided evidence that both FRC and CC are proportionately reduced with anesthesia.[27] These authors used the foreign gas bolus technique as opposed to the resident gas (N_2) technique used in the previous study and suggested that the latter might not adequately measure CC when lung volumes are restricted. However, an additional study found no difference when the two techniques were compared.[28] Therefore, the issue of whether awake control CC values are the same as those in anesthetized subjects is not resolved.

The degree of intrapulmonary shunting does appear to correlate with the reduction in FRC[29] and with the degree of atelectasis that develops in dependent lung regions.[30] It is thus tempting to attribute such atelectasis simply to the reduced FRC. However, a study in awake supine subjects with thoracoabdominal restriction argues against this simple mechanism.[31] The restriction in these subjects reduced lung volume and altered pulmonary mechanics in a fashion similar to that seen with general anesthesia. The FRC decreased by more than 20% and was matched by a reduction of CC as measured by the resident gas (N_2) technique. No atelectasis was noted with computed tomographic scanning, and ventilation-perfusion distribution and arterial blood gases were unchanged from the control state. Thus gas exchange in these awake subjects with chest restriction differed from that of anesthetized subjects, although both groups had the same relative decrement in FRC. The authors concluded that the development of compression atelectasis in the anesthetized patients cannot be ascribed solely to a decrease in FRC, nor can the changes in pulmonary mechanics with restriction be attributed solely to the development of atelectasis.

Intrapulmonary Gas Distribution

Ventilation is not normally uniform throughout the lung. The effects of gravity on the lung and the forces necessary to allow it to conform to the shape of the thorax result in a vertical gradient of pleural pressure.[32] The pleural pressure acting on the upper (nondependent) areas of the lung is more subatmospheric (negative) than that acting on the lower (dependent) portions. As a result, the nondependent areas are more inflated than the dependent ones (Fig. 8.4). The gradient of pleural pressure up and down the lung changes about 0.4 cm H_2O per each centimeter of lung height. Thus in a lung 30 cm high there is a pressure difference of 7.5 cm H_2O from apex to base. In the supine position the

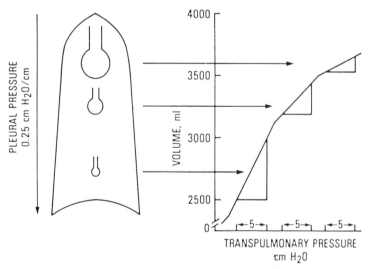

Figure 8.4.   The pleural pressure gradient increases down the lung so the dependent alveoli are small and the nondependent ones are relatively large. A change in transpulmonary pressure of 5 cm H_2O produces a greater change in volume (or ventilation) of the small dependent airspaces because they lie on a steeper portion of the compliance or pressure-volume curve. The large, nondependent alveoli lie on a flatter portion of the curve and thus undergo less volume change. (Reproduced with permission from Benumof JL. Respiration physiology and respiratory function during anesthesia. In: Miller RD, ed. Anesthesia. 3rd ed. New York: Churchill Livingstone, 1990:509.)

dorsal areas become dependent. The height of the lungs is reduced by nearly one-third and thus the gravitational effect is diminished somewhat.

Although the nondependent lung areas are more distended at FRC, a transpulmonary pressure of 5 cm generated during the normal breath produces a greater volume change or ventilation to the dependent areas. (Fig. 8.4). This is because of the sigmoid shape of the pressure-volume curve. The larger nondependent areas have a lower regional compliance; i.e., they lie on a less steep portion of the pressure-volume curve.

These regional differences in ventilation are important in matching ventilation to perfusion. The dependent or basal areas tend to be better perfused because of gravitational effects. Since the bases are also better ventilated there is good matching of ventilation and perfusion (Fig. 8.5). Higher ventilation and blood flow are delivered to the bases. In supine anesthetized paralyzed

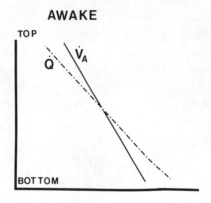

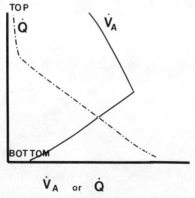

Figure 8.5. Diagrammatic representation of the distribution of ventilation ($\dot{V}_A$) and perfusion ($\dot{Q}$) between nondependent *(top)* lung areas and dependent *(bottom)* areas. Note that $\dot{V}_A$ tends to be distributed more uniformly from top to bottom in the anesthetized, paralyzed state. (Reproduced with permission from Gal TJ. Respiratory physiology during anesthesia. In: Kaplan JA, ed. Thoracic anesthesia. 2nd ed. New York: Churchill Livingstone, 1990, Chapter 8.)

humans, the ventilation or distribution of inspired gas becomes more uniform from top to bottom lung areas (Fig. 8.5), largely because basal lung units undergo further reduction in size to a point that reduces their regional compliance. Anesthetics, meanwhile, produce a decrease in pulmonary artery pressure that impedes perfusion on nondependent lung regions. Increased alveolar pressures with mechanical ventilation further interfere with perfusion of nondependent areas. Thus, dependent lung areas are well perfused but rather poorly ventilated. In contrast, nondependent areas receive more ventilation but considerably less perfusion.

The overall $\dot{V}A/\dot{Q}$ inhomogeneity may also be increased during anesthesia because of changes in airway caliber. The smooth muscle relaxation associated with anesthetics may be useful in preventing the increased bronchial tone associated with bronchospasm. However, reductions in normal bronchomotor tone may interfere with the normal ventilation-perfusion matching and thus impair gas exchange.[33]

In addition, local decreases in alveolar CO_2 tension tend to improve the normal ventilation-perfusion matching by producing local increases in bronchomotor tone. In a sense this hypocapneic bronchoconstriction is analogous to hypoxic pulmonary vasoconstriction. Whether or not the inhalation anesthetics as a group block this bronchoconstriction induced by hypocapnia is not known. Thus far only halothane has been shown to reduce this bronchoconstrictive effect of hypocapnia.[34,35]

Distribution of Ventilation in the Lateral Position

While lying in the lateral decubitus position subjects exhibit a greater blood flow to the dependent lung, largely because of gravitational effects. In the awake state the normal vertical gradient of pleural pressure also allows for greater ventilation of the same dependent lung and maintenance of normal ventilation-perfusion distribution. This is more true in the case of the larger right lung, which is not subject to compression by an enlarged heart. In fact, in relatively normal persons with unilateral lung disease, respiratory gas exchange is optimal if the good lung is dependent.[36,37] Exceptions to this appear to occur in infants and patients with chronic obstructive pulmonary disease, in whom the nondependent lung is better ventilated.[38,39]

Radiographic and bronchospirometric studies all show that the dependent lung normally receives a greater ventilation and has a higher O_2 uptake in the lateral position. Although its FRC is lower than that of the nondependent lung, N_2 washout is also more rapid.[40] When patients are anesthetized in the lateral position, as for thoracic surgery, distribution of the pulmonary blood flow is similar to the awake state; i.e., the dependent lung receives greater perfusion. A great portion of ventilation, however, is switched from the dependent to the nondependent lung. In a sense the ventilation is more uniform, and this is reflected in more equal N_2 clearance for each lung.[40] This shift in distribution of ventilation results from a loss of lung volume (decreased FRC), which is shared but unequally by both lungs. The dependent lung, which undergoes a greater decrease in FRC, moves to a less steep portion near the bottom of the pressure-volume curve (Fig. 8.4), while the nondependent lung moves from a relatively flat portion to a steeper one. The abdominal contents and the mediastinum also impede dependent lung expansion. Thus the anesthetized patient in the lateral position has a nondependent lung that is well ventilated but poorly perfused. In contrast, the well-perfused dependent lung is poorly ventilated. Opening the chest may only serve to increase the overventilation of the nondependent lung.

In summary, the increased ventilation-perfusion that accompanies anesthesia and paralysis whether in the supine or the lateral position appears to be largely a result of altered distribution of ventilation with a relative failure of intrapulmonary perfusion to adjust.[41] Although some of this failure of blood flow to adjust for the altered ventilation may relate to inhibition of hypoxic pulmonary vasoconstriction by the inhalation anesthetics, the altered pattern of expansion of the lung with anesthesia and paralysis may also affect the distribution of blood flow along with ventilation.

CLINICAL CONDITIONS ASSOCIATED WITH IMPAIRED GAS EXCHANGE

Pulmonary Edema

By far the most common clinical etiology of pulmonary edema is one in which the forces that drive fluid across the vessel wall are increased. Such increased intravascular pressures are the hallmark of cardiogenic pulmonary edema, i.e., that associated with congestive heart failure. Early in the development of pulmonary edema, well in advance of fluid accumulation in the airspace, interstitial fluid has been shown to accumulate around arterioles and bronchioles.[42] This "cuffing" action serves to increase both airway and pulmonary vascular resistance at the lung bases. Both ventilation and perfusion are redistributed away from these lower lung zones to more apical areas, and an imbalance in the ventilation-perfusion relationship results. The immediate consequence of this ventilation-perfusion mismatch is arterial hypoxemia, with average Pao_2 values of 50 to 55 mm Hg commonly observed.[43] Hypercapnia is not considered a usual consequence of pulmonary edema; however, elevated $Paco_2$ values have been reported.[43] The mechanism for hypercapnia is not entirely clear but may be related to the severity of the ventilation-perfusion imbalance.[4] Normally, hyperventilation can compensate for hypercapnia since the CO_2 dissociation curve is linear. However, if the work of breathing is significantly increased as with the congested stiff lung with increased airway resistance, ventilation may not be able to increase sufficiently to restore $Paco_2$ to normal. Furthermore, with extremely high work of breathing the metabolic load produced by the increased ventilation may offset the exhaled CO_2 and worsen hypercapnia.

Other noncardiac varieties of pulmonary edema basically consist of a condition in which fluid movement to the outside of vessels is increased because of increased permeability, usually from loss of the integrity of the vessel wall. This group includes such states as the adult respiratory distress syndrome, neurogenic pulmonary edema, and the pulmonary edema associated with heroin overdose or exposure to high altitude. The major abnormality of gas exchange in such patients results from large degrees of intrapulmonary shunting. The arterial hypoxemia in these states is also quite vulnerable to any factors that alter $P\bar{v}o_2$, in particular cardiac output.

One other variant of pulmonary edema with transient failure of gas exchange in the form of an increased alveolar-arterial O_2 difference is that associated with the development and relief of acute upper airway obstruction. Many factors play a role in the pathogenesis of such pulmonary edema. However, the fact that it is often referred to as "negative-pressure pulmonary edema" simplistically implies that a marked negative inspiratory pressure is the predominant if not the only cause. Lloyd et al.[44] demonstrated that negative inspiratory pressures associated with breathing through inspiratory resistances promoted lung lymph formation in sheep in a fashion similar to that resulting from elevated intravascular pressures. On the other hand, Hansen et al.[45] were unable to show any effect of inspiratory obstruction on steady-state lung lymph flow. Since the latter study used supplemental O_2 the authors postulated that a key to the development of edema is the presence of alveolar hypoxia, which mediates pulmonary vasoconstriction and may cause capillary leak. This is an attractive explanation, since patients with upper airway obstruction are usually not receiving O_2 and are likely to experience severe hypoxia. Other interesting evidence that has cast some doubt on the dominant role of negative pressure in the genesis of pulmonary edema is the abundance of studies in which human subjects[46] or animals[47] have breathed against severe extrinsic inspiratory obstructions and developed inspiratory pressures more than 10 times those of quiet breathing and yet have not developed pulmonary edema.

Pulmonary Embolism

Abnormal gas exchange inevitably accompanies acute pulmonary embolism. Abnormalities are influenced by the size and extent of the vascular occlusion, the presence of underlying cardiovascular disease, and the time since the acute embolization. Arterial hypoxemia is frequently though not universally found. However, the patients in whom significant arterial hypoxemia does not develop with ambient air (Pao_2 80 mm Hg) do exhibit an increased alveolar to arterial oxygen gradient. The failure of these patients to develop hypoxemia results from the hyperventilation that usually accompanies the embolism. In most of these patients the increased ventilation is associated with some hypocapnia.

The other most significant consequence of the embolism is an increased alveolar dead space, because the occlusion is associated with absent flow to distal lung areas. The occlusion may not be total and thus regions of high $\dot{V}_A/\dot{Q}$ ratios may prevail. These zones of lung with vascular obstruction develop "pneumoconstriction," which may be the result of both airway hypocapnia and the release of bronchoconstrictive amines.

This pneumoconstriction teleologically reduces the extent of the alveolar dead space and high $\dot{V}_A/\dot{Q}$ areas but may contribute to the development of low $\dot{V}_A/\dot{Q}$ zones. Such zones may preexist in many patients. They also can increase acutely from hyperperfusion of the vascular bed in unaffected areas and from the development of atelectasis distal to areas of vascular obstruction.

Another important contributor to the abnormal oxygenation is a reduction in cardiac output because of right ventricular failure. This generally requires massive vascular obstruction ($>50\%$). As cardiac output falls $P\bar{v}_{O_2}$ is also decreased and amplifies the effect of right-to-left shunting and low $\dot{V}_A/\dot{Q}$ areas.[48]

Bronchospasm

Episodes of bronchoconstriction in asthmatics, whether spontaneous or induced by bronchial provocation testing, are associated not only with increased airflow resistance but also with changes in gas exchange. The most prominent manifestation is hypoxemia, and most current evidence points to ventilation-perfusion abnormalities as the major cause. There appears to be a marked broadening of ventilation-perfusion relationships with a preponderance of very low but finite $\dot{V}_A/\dot{Q}$ ratios but no absolute shunt.[49]

Inhalation of aerosolized isoproterenol is associated with worsening of hypoxemia and ventilation-perfusion inequality, presumably from an increased perfusion of lung units with low $\dot{V}_A/\dot{Q}$ ratios. This apparent decrease in pulmonary vascular resistance and increased perfusion of low $\dot{V}_A/\dot{Q}$ areas suggests that isoproterenol may be inhibiting hypoxic pulmonary vasoconstriction (HPV). However, this may not be the entire mechanism, since breathing pure oxygen does not seem to increase flow to these low $\dot{V}_A/\dot{Q}$ areas.[49]

Patients with severe acute asthma requiring mechanical ventilation exhibit qualitatively the same pattern of ventilation-perfusion abnormalities seen in less severe disease. They do, however, have a high degree of preexisting HPV, which responds to breathing pure oxygen with a significant amount of shunt.[50] While the latter may also reflect the development of absorption atelectasis,[51] it is most likely due to increased perfusion of these previously insignificant shunt areas.

Pulmonary Aspiration of Gastric Contents

The initial response to the aspiration of acidic gastric contents is one of intense bronchoconstriction. This irritative reaction is rapidly followed by transudation of large amounts of fluid from the respiratory epithelium into the airspaces. The result is profound arterial hypoxemia ($Pao_2 < 50$), as in severe cardiogenic pulmonary edema. Increased Fio_2 offsets the hypoxemia, but a large alveolar-arterial O_2 difference persists as a reflection of the severe ventilation-perfusion mismatch. As in cardiogenic pulmonary edema, this mismatch may be severe enough, given the increased work of breathing, to also impair CO_2 removal. The degree of respiratory acidosis depends on the ability to produce adequate alveolar ventilation, while metabolic acidosis may result from concomitant tissue hypoxia.

Pneumothorax

The clinical presentation of pneumothorax may be confused with bronchospasm because of the presence of increased airway pressure, wheezing, diminshed breath sounds, and hypoxemia. This is further complicated by the fact that pneumothorax is more frequent in patients with obstructive airway disease. Progressive expansion of the pneumothorax compresses lung parenchyma and creates more and more areas with low $\dot{V}A/\dot{Q}$ ratios, and thus hypoxemia. The limited ability to increase ventilation and the cardiac depression may be associated with hypercapnia as well.

INFLUENCE OF DISEASE STATES ON GAS EXCHANGE

Cardiac Disease

Cardiac function has its most obvious effect on gas exchange via its effect on the oxygen content of mixed venous blood. If cardiac function is inadequate to match the demands of peripheral O_2 delivery, arterial-venous O_2 differences increase and have an eventual effect on Pao_2. Mild degrees of cardiac failure, in contrast to the already discussed effects of pulmonary edema, are associated with minimal effects on gas exchange and little or no alteration in ventilation-perfusion distributions.

Renal Disease

Patients with renal disease often exhibit hypocapnia as a result of attempts to compensate for systemic acidosis by hyperventilation. The presence of coexistent lung disease or cardiac failure may result in hypoxemia. Arterial hypoxemia is also commonly observed during and after hemodialysis. Both the acetate and bicarbonate dialysates are associated with hypoxemia, which appears to be related to a transitory hypoventilation.[52] The acetate removes some of the CO_2 load presented, while with bicarbonate dialysis it appears that respiratory drive is suppressed by a gain in bicarbonate. Ventilation-perfusion abnormalities appear to contribute somewhat to this postdialysis hypoxemia, which is similar in patients with and without lung disease.[53] Another contributing factor may be the reduction in cardiac output that so commonly occurs with dialysis.[54] However, the principal cause of the reduced arterial O_2 tension appears to be a decrease in alveolar O_2 tension (Pao_2) because of hypoventilation.[55] Thus the $AaDo_2$ does not change and Pao_2 is reduced concomitantly with Pao_2. This is somewhat analogous to the posthyperventilation hypoxia described following general anesthesia.[56]

Liver Disease

In patients with hepatic cirrhosis who have relatively normal lung mechanics, arterial hypoxemia is a frequent finding. In patients with mild hypoxemia the abnormal gas exchange is primarily due to ventilation-perfusion mismatch.[57] Patients with severe hypoxemia have exhibited considerable right-to-left shunting as well.[58] Clinically, such patients demonstrate decreased oxygenation in the upright compared to the recumbent position (orthodeoxia) as well as dyspnea in the upright position that is relieved by recumbency (platypnea).

Obesity

The reduced respiratory system compliance and other mechanical ventilatory consequences of obesity would predict that abnormal gas exchange is likely. Indeed, hypoxemia, usually unaccompanied by hypercapnia, is present. This is most likely a reflection of closed peripheral lung units of low $\dot{V}a/\dot{Q}$ ratios and increased shunting.[59]

Of considerable importance are the added derangements of cardiovascular and respiratory function imposed by changes in posture in the obese patient.[60] Movement from the upright to the recumbent and Trendelenburg positions would have progressively more adverse consequences on lung volumes and oxygenation during and after anesthesia. In the immediate postoperative period, for example, the semirecumbent position seems to be associated with better oxygenation than the supine position.[61]

Pulmonary Disease

Restrictive Disease.   The common element in the many forms of restrictive pulmonary disease is a loss of lung volume. This is a result of alterations in one of the major structural components of the thorax: skeletal, neuromuscular, pleural, or lung parenchyma (interstitial and alveolar). The reduction in lung volume is associated with a decreased lung compliance, the major consequences of which are increased work of breathing and maldistribution of ventilation. This maldistribution produces low $\dot{V}a/\dot{Q}$ areas whose major impact on arterial blood gases is a pattern of hypoxemia, hypocapnia, and an increase in AaD_{O_2}. The hypocapnia indicates that hyperventilation is effective in maintaining CO_2 excretion. If hypercapnia occurs, it usually indicates advanced terminal disease in restrictive illness.

Obstructive Disease. Chronic obstructive disease spans the spectrum between airflow obstruction (bronchitis) and overinflation or air trapping (emphysema). The maldistribution of ventilation that impairs gas exchange results from abnormally long time constants (R × C). In the case of bronchitis resistance (R) is increased, while compliance (C) is increased in emphysema. In emphysematous patients ("pink puffers") high $\dot{V}A/\dot{Q}$ areas or areas of relatively "wasted ventilation" are prominent. Such patients tend to exhibit some mild hypoxemia and are usually normocapneic despite high levels of resting ventilation. In contrast, the more bronchitic types ("blue bloaters") characteristically exhibit more low $\dot{V}A/\dot{Q}$ areas and present with moderate to severe hypoxemia ($Pa_{O_2} < 50$ mm Hg) and significant hypercapnia ($Pa_{CO_2} > 50$ mm Hg).

REFERENCES

1. Askenazi J, Weissman C, Rosenbaum SH, Hyman AI, Milic-Emili J, Kinney JM. Nutrition and the respiratory system. Crit Care Med 1982;10:163–172.
2. Kaplan JA, Bush GL, Lecky JH, Ominsy AJ, Wollman H. Sodium bicarbonate and systemic hemodynamics in volunteers anesthetized with halothane. Anesthesiology 1975;42:550–558.
3. Shepard RH, Campbell EJM, Martin HB, Enns T. Factors affecting the pulmonary dead space as determined by single breath analysis. J Appl Physiol 1975;11:241–244.
4. West JB. Causes of carbon dioxide retention in lung disease. N Engl J Med 1971;284:1232–1236.
5. Figueras J, Stein L, Diez V, Weil MH, Shobin H. Relationships between pulmonary hemodynamics and arterial pH and carbon dioxide tension in critically ill patients. Chest 1976;70:460–472.
6. Juan G, Calverley P, Talamo C, Schnader J, Roussos C. Effect of carbon dioxide on diaphragmatic function in human beings. N Engl J Med 1984;310:874–879.
7. Edwards R, Winnie AP, Ramamurthy S. Acute hypocapneic hypokalemia; an iatrogenic anesthetic complication. Anesth Analg 1977;46:786–792.
8. Cutillo A, Omboni E, Perondi R, Tana F. Effect of hypocapnia on pulmonary mechanics in normal subjects and in patients with chronic obstructive pulmonary disease. Am Rev Respir Dis 1974;110:25–33.
9. Nunn JF. Applied respiratory physiology. 3rd ed. Boston: Butterworths, 1987:227–228.
10. Eger EI, Severinghaus J. The rate of rise of P_ACO_2 in the apneic anesthetized patient. Anesthesiology 1961;22:419–425.
11. Chiang ST. A nomogram for venous shunt ($\dot{Q}s/\dot{Q}t$) calculation. Thorax 1968;23:563–565.
12. Torda TA. Alveolar-arterial oxygen tensions difference: a critical look. Anaesth Intensive Care 1981;9:326–330.
13. VanDeWater JM, Kagey HS, Miller IT, et al. Response of the lung to six to twelve hours of one hundred percent oxygen. N Engl J Med 1970;283:621–626.
14. Mithoefer JC, Keighley JF, Karetzky MS. Response of the arterial Po_2 to oxygen administration in chronic pulmonary disease. Ann Intern Med 1971;74:328–335.
15. Gilbert R, Keighley JF. The arterial/alveolar oxygen tension ratio. An index of gas exchange applicable to varying inspired oxygen concentrations. Am Rev Respir Dis 1974;109:142–145.
16. Zetterstrom H. Assessment of the efficiency of pulmonary oxygenation. The choice of oxygenation index. Acta Anaesthesiol Scand 1988;32:579–584.
17. Siegel JH, Farrel EJ. A computer simulation model to study the clinical observability of ventilation and perfusion abnormalities in human shock states. Surgery 1973;73:898–912.

18. Hegyi T, Hiatt M. Respiratory index: a simple evaluation of the severity of idiopathic respiratory distress syndrome. Crit Care Med 1979;7:500–501.

19. Wagner PD, Saltzman HA, West JB. Measurement of continuous distributions of ventilation-perfusion ratios: theory. J Appl Physiol 1974;36:588–599.

20. Teplick RM, Snider MT, Gilbert JP. A comparison of continuous and discrete foreign gas $\dot{V}_A/\dot{Q}$ distributions. J Appl Physiol 1980;49:684–692.

21. Hlastala MP. Multiple inert gas eliminations technique. J Appl Physiol 1984;56:1–7.

22. Dueck R, Young I, Clausen J, Wagner PD. Altered distribution of pulmonary ventilation and blood flow following induction of inhalational anesthesia. Anesthesiology 1980;52:113–125.

23. Rehder K, Marsh HYM, Rodare JR, Hyatt RE. Airway closure. Anesthesiology 1977;47:40–52.

24. Hickey RF, Visick WD, Fairley HB, Fourcade HE. Effects of halothane anesthesia on functional residual capacity and alveolar-arterial oxygen tension difference. Anesthesiology 1973;38:20–24.

25. Gilmour J, Burnham M, Crag DG. Closing capacity measurement during general anesthesia. Anesthesiology 1976;45:477–482.

26. Hedensteirna G, McCartha G, Bergstrom M. Airway closure during mechanical ventilation. Anesthesiology 1976;44:114–123.

27. Juno P, Marsh HM, Knopp TJ, Rehder K. Closing capacity in awake and anesthetized paralyzed man. J Appl Physiol 1978;44:238–244.

28. Hedenstierna G, Santesson J. Airway closure during anesthesia: a comparison between resident gas and argon bolus techniques. J Appl Physiol 1979;47:874–881.

29. Dueck R, Prutow RJ, Davies NJH, Clausen JL, Davidson TM. The lung volume at which shunting occurs with inhalation anesthesia. Anesthesiology 1988;69:854–861.

30. Hedenstierna G, Tokics L, Strandberg A, Lundquist H, Brismar B. Correlation of gas exchange impairment to development of atelectasis during anesthesia and muscle paralysis. Acta Anaesthesiol Scand 1986;30:183–191.

31. Tokics L, Hedenstierna G, Brismar B, Strandberg A. Thoracoabdominal restriction in supine man: CT and lung function measurements. J Appl Physiol 1988;64:599–604.

32. Agostoni E. Mechanics of the pleural space. Physiol Rev 1972;52:57–128.

33. Crawford ABH, Makowska M, Engel LA. Effect of bronchomotor tone on static mechanical properties of lung and ventilation distribution. J Appl Physiol 1987;63:2278–2285.

34. McAsian C, Mima M, Norden I, Norlander O. Effects of halothane and methoxyflurane on pulmonary resistance to gas flow during lung bypass. Scand J Thorac Cardiovasc Surg 1971;5:193–197.

35. Coon RL, Kampine JP. Hypocapneic bronchoconstriction and inhalation anesthetics. Anesthesiology 1975;43:635–641.

36. Remolina C, Kahn AU, Santiago TV, Edelman NH. Positional hypoxemia in unilateral lung disease. N Engl J Med 1981;304:523–525.

37. Fishman AF. Down with the good lung. N Engl J Med 1981;304:537–538.

38. Dvies H, Kitchman R, Gordon I, Helms P. Regional ventilation in infancy. Reversal of adult pattern. N Engl J Med 1985;313:1626–1628.

39. Shim C, Chun K, Williams MH, Blaufox MD. Positional effects on distribution of ventilation in chronic obstructive pulmonary disease. Ann Intern Med 1986;105:346–350.

40. Rehder K, Hatch, Sessler AD, Fowler WS. The function of each lung of anesthetized paralyzed man during mechanical ventilation. Anesthesiology 1972;37:16–26.

41. Landmark SJ, Knopp TJ, Rehder K, Sessler AD. Regional pulmonary perfusion and $\dot{V}/\dot{Q}$ in awake and anesthetized paralyzed man. J Appl Physiol 1977;43:993–1000.

42. Staub NE, Nagand H, Pearch ML. Pulmonary edema in dogs, especially the sequence of fluid accumulation in lungs. J Appl Physiol 1967;22:227–240.

43. Aberman AD, Fulop M. The metabolic and respiratory acidosis of acute pulmonary edema. Ann Intern Med 1972;76:173–184.

44. Lloyd JE, Nolop KB, Parker RE, Roselli RJ, Brigham KL. Effects of inspiratory resistance loading on lung fluid balance in awake sheep. J Appl Physiol 1986;60:198–203.

45. Hansen TN, Gest AL, Landers S. Inspiratory airway obstruction does not affect lung fluid balance in lambs. J Appl Physiol 1985;58:1314–1318.

46. Roussos CS, Macklem PT. Diaphragmatic fatigue in man. J Appl Physiol 1977;43:189–197.

47. Bazzy AR, Haddad GG. Diaphragmatic fatigue in unanesthetized adult sheep. J Appl Physiol 1984;57:182–190.
48. D'Alonzo GE, Dantzker DR. Gas exchange alterations following pulmonary thromboembolism. Clin Chest Med 1984;5:411–419.
49. Wagner PD, Dantzger DR, Iacovoni VE, Tomlin WC, West JB. Ventilation perfusion inequality in asymptomatic asthma. Am Rev Respir Dis 1978;118:511–524.
50. Rodriguez-Roisin R, Ballester E, Roca J, Torres A, Wagner PD. Mechanisms of hypoxemia in patients with status asthmaticus requiring mechanical ventilation. Am Rev Respir Dis 1989;139:732–739.
51. Dantzger DR, Wagner PD, West JB. Instability of lung units with low $\dot{V}_A/\dot{Q}$ ratios during O_2 breathing. J Appl Physiol 1975;38:886–895.
52. Hunt JM, Chappel TR, Henrich WL, Rubin LJ. Gas exchange during dialysis. Am J Med 1984;77:255–260.
53. Pitcher WD, Diamond SM, Henrich WL. Pulmonary gas exchange during dialysis in patients with obstructive lung disease. Chest 1989;96:1136–1141.
54. Handt A, Farber MO, Szwed JJ. Intradialytic measurement of cardiac output by thermodilution and impedance cardiography. Clin Nephrol 1977;7:61–64.
55. Patterson RW, Nissenson AR, Miller J, Smith RT, Narins RO, Sullivan SF. Hypoxemia and pulmonary gas exchange during hemodialysis. J Appl Physiol 1981;50:259–264.
56. Sullivan SF, Patterson RW, Papper EM. Post hyperventilation hypoxia. J Appl Physiol 1967;22:431–435.
57. Melot C, Naeije R, Dechamps P, Hallemans R, Lejeune P. Pulmonary and extrapulmonary contributors to hypoxemia in liver cirrhosis. Am Rev Respir Dis 1989;139:632–640.
58. Edell EJ, Cortese OP, Krowka MJ, Redher K. Severe hypoxemia and liver disease. Am Rev Respir Dis 1989;140:1631–1635.
59. Rochester DF, Enson Y. Current concepts in the pathogenesis of obesity-hypoventilation syndrome; mechanical and circulatory factors. Am J Med 1974;57:402–420.
60. Paul DR, Hoyt JL, Boutros AR. Cardiovascular and respiratory changes in response to change of posture in the very obese. Anesthesiology 1976;45:73–78.
61. Vaughn RW, Wise L. Postoperative arterial blood gas measurement: effect of position on gas exchange. Ann Surg 1975;182:705–709.

Physiology of Mechanical Ventilation and Applied Airway Pressure

Chapter 9

Basic Concepts of Ventilation

FORCES INVOLVED IN PRODUCING AIRFLOW

For air to flow into and out of the lungs, the respiratory system (lungs and chest wall) must first expand and then return to a resting volume. Sufficient force must be developed to overcome the elastic recoil and flow resistance of the respiratory system. Normally such force is provided by contraction of the respiratory muscles. Their action produces a subatmospheric pressure in the airways and thus a pressure gradient between the airways and the mouth. This gradient is responsible for airflow into the lungs. As inspiration ceases, expiration, a purely passive activity, begins. The energy stored in the elastic recoil of the lungs and chest wall produces an increase in alveolar pressure such that the pressure gradient is reversed and air is forced out of the lungs.

Mechanical devices can be utilized to apply this subatmospheric pressure around the patient's entire body (iron lungs) or only around the chest wall (cuirass ventilators). Although such negative-pressure ventilators are sometimes used to support patients with neuromuscular weakness, ventilatory support is usually provided by positive-pressure ventilators, which generate a pressure greater than atmospheric pressure to force air into the alveoli. In either case lung expansion is a function of changes in transpulmonary pressure (P_L), which reflects the difference between alveolar pressure (P_A) and pleural pressure (Ppl), i.e., $P_L = P_A - Ppl$. In spontaneous or negative-pressure ventilation, Pl and hence lung volume are increased by a decrease (more negative) in Ppl (Fig. 9.1**A**). With conventional mechanical ventilation P_L is increased, but instead by an increase in P_A (Fig. 9.1**B**).

PHYSIOLOGIC EFFECTS OF INCREASED AIRWAY PRESSURE

Among physiologists the Valsalva and Mueller maneuvers have been time-honored techniques for studying the effects of positive and negative pressure on the circulation. The Valsalva maneuver consists of an expiratory effort in the presence of a closed glottis, while the Mueller maneuver is an inspiratory effort

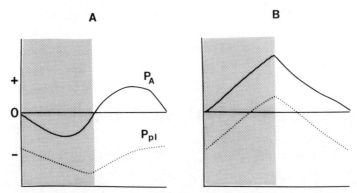

Figure 9.1.   Diagrammatic illustration of changes in airway or alveolar pressure (P_A) and pleural pressure (Ppl) during spontaneous (**A**) and mechanical (**B**) ventilation. The *shaded areas* indicate the period of inspiration.

against a closed glottis. During a Valsalva maneuver the volume of blood returning to the thorax decreases, while the Mueller maneuver results in an increase in the volume of blood returning. Although these two situations produce hemodynamic alterations similar to positive- and negative-pressure breathing, the effects on lung inflation differ. In the case of the Valsalva and Mueller maneuvers, lung volume does not change. This is because P_L does not change, i.e., P_A and Ppl change to the same extent.

Mean Airway Pressure

The instantaneous positive pressure applied to the airway varies during each respiratory cycle (Fig. 9.1**B**). The physiologic effects of such pressure depend not only on the instantaneous magnitude of the pressure but also on the length of time it is applied to the airway. A clinically useful composite of all the pressures transmitted to the airway during mechanical ventilation is the mean airway pressure ($\overline{P}aw$), or the average pressure present in the airways. The $\overline{P}aw$ can be thought of simply as the area under the pressure curve. This can be estimated graphically (Fig. 9.2) or by electronic integration of the signal from a pressure transducer. In either case $\overline{P}aw$ is computed by dividing the area under the pressure curve by the total time for each respiratory cycle.

Many factors influence the values for $\overline{P}aw$. Perhaps the most obvious is the deliberate use of high driving pressures or excessive volumes to ventilate. Prolongation of the inspiratory time also increases $\overline{P}aw$, since the inspiratory portion of the pressure curve has the largest area per unit time (Fig. 9.2).

Essentially the area under the pressure curve varies directly with the duration of inspiration and inversely with the length of expiration. Thus any increase in the ratio of inspiratory time to expiratory time (I:E ratio) will increase $\overline{P}aw$ if the total respiratory cycle is unchanged. One such prolongation of inspiration occurs with an end-inspiratory pause in which the lungs are

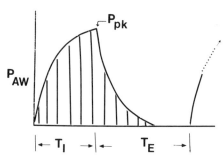

Figure 9.2. Graphic representation of airway pressure (Paw) tracing during a respiratory cycle, which consists of inspiration (Tı) and expiration (Tᴇ). Mean airway pressure can be estimated by measuring the length of each line from the dots on the pressure curve to zero pressure and dividing by their sums by the number of measurements. Ppk, peak airway pressure.

held inflated at a fixed level of pressure or volume for a time. The longer this time, the greater the area under the pressure curve and the higher the $\overline{P}$aw.

Expiratory resistance or "retard" has been employed in mechanical ventilation to mimic pursed-lips breathing with the hopes of allowing more uniform lung emptying. The technique involves placement of a variable resistance in the exhalation circuit to slow expiratory flow. Thus expiratory pressures decrease more slowly and contribute to increasing $\overline{P}$aw.

Positive end-expiratory pressure (PEEP), which is discussed in more detail later in this chapter, is a maneuver in which airway pressure is not allowed to decrease to atmospheric pressure at the end of exhalation. The elevated baseline pressure that results with PEEP also contributes to an increased $\overline{P}$aw. Conversely, if negative pressure were applied during exhalation to produce negative end-expiratory pressure, $\overline{P}$aw would decrease.

The importance of $\overline{P}$aw has long been recognized in both laboratory[1] and clinical settings.[2] There appears to be a significant relationship between $\overline{P}$aw and the efficiency of oxygenation. The $\overline{P}$aw for adequate oxygenation increases as the severity of lung pathology intensifies and may be associated with an increased incidence of barotrauma. It is often difficult, however, to ascertain whether the barotrauma results from the absolute effects of increased $\overline{P}$aw or from the underlying pulmonary pathology.

Positive End-Expiratory Pressure

Positive end-expiratory pressure (PEEP) is a term that refers to any increase in airway pressure above atmospheric at end exhalation. Continuous positive-pressure breathing is not a new concept, having been introduced into medicine and used in aviation for more than 30 years. To understand and appreciate the physiologic consequences of PEEP, an understanding of the static elastic behavior of the respiratory system is essential (see Chapter 1). The respiratory system has two elastic components, the lung and the chest wall. Each has its position of equilibrium. The equilibrium position of the respiratory system occurs at the volume at which the tendency of the lung to recoil inward is offset by the outward recoil of the chest wall. This relaxation volume or functional residual capacity (FRC) in normal seated subjects occurs at 40 to 50% of total lung capacity (TLC).

Normally, exhalation is passive and occurs because of the recoil of the lung. At end expiration (FRC), alveolar pressure returns to zero (atmospheric). Any maneuver that does not allow the pressure to return to zero results in PEEP. Thus, expiratory flow ceases and end-expiratory volume occurs above FRC.

The PEEP can be applied by a number of devices, most of which are either threshold resistors or orifice resistors.[3] The threshold resistors exert a constant, predictable force that opposes pressures developed during exhalation. They consist of water columns, weighted ball valves that are gravity dependent, and spring-loaded valves that are not gravity dependent. With orifice resistors the pressures developed are the result of the product of flow ($\dot{V}$) and the resistance (R) of the device. Since R is fixed, the pressure is directly related to $\dot{V}$. The orifice resistors therefore are totally dependent on $\dot{V}$ to maintain PEEP. If $\dot{V}$ is too low in the presence of an orifice resistor, the system will function as an expiratory resistance or retard and will not develop true PEEP. On the other hand, the relatively high expiratory flow rates achievable by adults may result in dangerously high PEEP levels. For this reason such flow-resistive devices are limited to small pediatric patients.

Cardiorespiratory Effects of PEEP.   The prime reason for using PEEP is to improve oxygenation in patients who are dangerously hypoxemic in spite of a high FIO_2. The beneficial effects appear to be related to the increased lung volume. Distal conducting airways and already patent alveoli undergo distention, which prevents their collapse during expiration and promotes recruitment of previously collapsed airways. This passive mechanical distention appears to be similar with PEEP (which is the term used by convention when positive end-expiratory pressure is applied during mechanical ventilation) and with continuous positive airway pressure (CPAP) applied during spontaneous ventilation.[4]

The ability of PEEP therapy to improve oxygenation in pulmonary edema, whether of the cardiogenic or noncardiogenic (increased permeability) variety, led to the hypothesis that extravascular lung water might be decreased by PEEP. However, most studies have shown that the improved oxygenation is not associated with decreased extravascular lung water.[5,6] Rather, morphometric data suggest that PEEP is associated with a redistribution of lung water from the alveoli to perivascular areas where the impact on gas exchange is lessened.[7]

The increased functioning lung volume that occurs as a result of alveolar recruitment improves gas exchange. Shunt or venous admixture is decreased because of improved ventilation-perfusion relationships. Areas of low ventilation perfusion ($\dot{V}A/\dot{Q}$) ratios are converted to those with more optimal $\dot{V}A/$

$\dot{Q}$ ratios, while others are converted to regions with a high $\dot{V}A$ relative to $\dot{Q}$. The development of such high $\dot{V}A/\dot{Q}$ regions, which behave functionally like dead space, appears to be due to redistribution of pulmonary blood flow and not of $\dot{V}A$. This impact on pulmonary perfusion reflects the adverse effects of PEEP on cardiac output and pulmonary vascular resistance, both of which reduce the effectiveness of PEEP in increasing PaO_2. Cardiac output may be reduced because of hypovolemia or cardiac disease. In the former case, cardiac filling pressures are reduced. Cardiac output may also be reduced because of transmission of airway pressure to the pulmonary vasculature, in particular alveolar vessels. In patients with normal lungs, applied pressure causes the lungs to expand. As a result, pleural pressures become more positive and compress veins in the thorax to impede venous return. Pulmonary vascular resistance also increases because alveolar vessels are compressed. Thus, right heart output should be decreased by diminished venous return and by increased right ventricular afterload in the form of elevated pulmonary vascular resistance. At least this is what seems intuitively obvious. Nevertheless, data from healthy volunteers during positive-pressure ventilation with 10 cm H_2O PEEP[8] demonstrated a 20% fall in cardiac output, but transmural right atrial pressure rose 3 cm H_2O, and right ventricular diastolic size increased 15%; left ventricular size decreased 20%. Thus, right ventricular filling did not appear to be significantly decreased. Rather, left ventricular filling decreased.

In the presence of pulmonary edema and decreased lung compliance, there is less lung distention with PEEP and pleural pressure does not rise appreciably to reduce venous return. However, pulmonary vascular resistance is increased because of compression of alveolar vessels by the high alveolar pressure. Thus, the decreased cardiac output caused by pressure breathing under these circumstances is due mostly to pulmonary vascular resistance caused by compression of alveolar vessels.[9] However, because of the relatively small changes in lung volume, pulmonary vascular resistance is elevated less than in normal subjects and cardiac output is usually less affected.

In summary, although the cardiorespiratory effects of PEEP are not entirely understood, at least three factors may contribute to the decrease in cardiac output.[10] These include, first, some decreased venous return with a resultant decrease in right ventricular filling. More important, there is an increased right ventricular afterload secondary to increased pulmonary vascular resistance. Finally, left ventricular end-diastolic dimensions are decreased. The latter is a function of reduced ventricular distensibility and filling with no associated impairment of contractility. Each of these factors requires a separate strategy for correcting the adverse hemodynamic consequences of PEEP.

PRINCIPLES OF MECHANICAL VENTILATION

The basic operation of a mechanical ventilator consists of inflating the lung to a certain point, ceasing the inflation, allowing the lungs to deflate, and then initiating another respiratory cycle by once again inflating the lungs. This process can be analyzed in four separate phases to understand the function of any ventilator.[11]

1. Inspiratory phase
2. Transition from inspiration to expiration
3. Expiratory phase
4. Transition from expiration to inspiration

Inspiratory Phase

To initiate inspiration a positive-pressure ventilator must develop a pressure differential between the proximal airway and the alveoli. Important factors to consider during the inspiratory phase include the tidal volume (VT) or the volume of gas delivered, the rate at which it is delivered (inspiratory flow), the pressure in the system required to deliver the volume, and finally the pressure that develops in the airways or alveoli once the volume of gas is delivered.

During inspiration the volume of gas delivered (VT) is essentially a function of inspiratory gas flow ($\dot{V}I$) over a period referred to as the inspiratory time (TI). Two basic mechanisms are utilized by mechanical ventilators to deliver VT such that they may be classified as flow generators or pressure generators. When a ventilator produces a $\dot{V}I$ pattern that is consistent regardless of increasing airway pressure (Paw) it is referred to as a flow generator (Fig. 9.3**A**). In addition to this constant "square wave" $\dot{V}I$ pattern, a flow generator may develop a nonconstant flow pattern, the most common of which is a sinusoidal wave (Fig. 9.3**B**). However, accelerating (Fig. 9.3**C**) and decelerating (Fig. 9.3**D**) patterns may also be utilized.

A ventilator that produces a sustained, relatively uniform pressure throughout inspiration is referred to as a constant-pressure generator. Gas

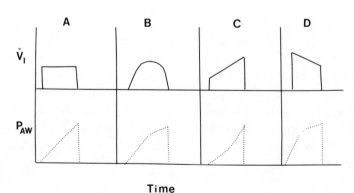

Figure 9.3.   Patterns for inspiratory flow ($\dot{V}I$) and airway pressure (Paw) developed with four mechanical ventilators that function as flow generators. **A**, Constant ("square-wave") flow pattern. **B**, Nonconstant (sinusoidal). **C**, Accelerating flow. **D**, Decelerating flow.

flow from such a ventilator reaches its maximum early in inspiration when the gradient between applied pressure and the alveolar pressure in the patient's lung is greatest. As pressure within the patient's airways increases, flow decreases toward zero as the airway pressure approaches the driving pressure. The resultant $\dot{V}I$ pattern is one of decelerating flow (Fig. 9.4**A**). Pressure generators may also be nonconstant, i.e., develop a changing (increasing) pressure during inspiration (Fig. 9.4**B**). As Paw increases, flow also decreases but in a slower, less uniform, exponential fashion as with constant pressure.

Both types of pressure generators are used primarily for short-term ventilators, since the delivered tidal volume is a function of the pressure applied but is highly dependent on the resistance and compliance of the patient's respiratory system. For the most part the ventilators used on anesthesia machines tend to be of the constant-flow generator type. If the driving or working pressure for such ventilators is high enough, there will be little difference between $\dot{V}I$ at the beginning and the end of inspiration, and thus a true square-wave pattern would result. As the circuit pressure rises and approaches the driving pressure, the $\dot{V}I$ delivered by the ventilator tends to decrease appreciably. Thus, rather than a square wave, the $\dot{V}I$ pattern is likely to be one of decelerating flow, which may limit delivery of adequate VT. The mean inspiratory flow may also decrease with increased Paw because of gas compression and distensibility of the breathing circuit and ventilator bellows.

A number of critical care ventilators (e.g., Siemens Servo 900D), because of their high working pressure, are able to maintain constant flows at Paw levels as high as 80 cm H_2O. The $\dot{V}I$ is maintained because of the small compressible volume within the ventilator and a flow generator that is pressure independent

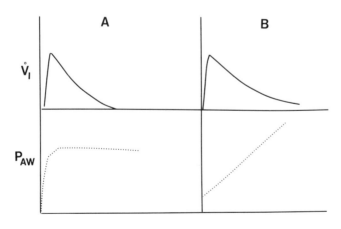

Figure 9.4.   Inspiratory flow $\dot{V}I$ and airway pressure (Paw) patterns developed by two examples of pressure-generator ventilators. **A,** Constant-pressure generator. **B,** Nonconstant-pressure generator.

until its preset working pressure limit is reached. The advantages of such a ventilator have been demonstrated in a lung model[12] and may apply to a limited number of patients with acute respiratory failure who require anesthesia.

Inspiratory Flow Rates.   Most ventilators deliver inspiratory flow rates ($\dot{V}I$) over a range of 10 liters/min up to 120 liters/min (i.e., 2 liters/sec). Flow rates of 60 liters/min (1 liter/sec) are common settings for average adults. This $\dot{V}I$ corresponds to the flow rates associated with a normal deep breath, and $\dot{V}I$ levels below this may be associated with sensations of dyspnea in awake, ventilated patients. It is also important to note that such ventilator settings usually refer to square-wave flow patterns in which the mean and peak $\dot{V}I$ values are essentially the same. If other patterns such as sinusoidal accelerating or decelerating flows are used, the setting usually refers to peak $\dot{V}I$. This is an important distinction, since it is the mean $\dot{V}I$, not the peak, that along with VT settings determines the duration of inspiration (TI).

Inspiratory flow rates are very important determinants not only of TI but also of peak inspiratory pressure. More important, $\dot{V}I$ may also influence the distribution of ventilation throughout the lung. During a normal slow inspiration gas flow is preferentially distributed to the more compliant basal or dependent lung regions. During a fast inspiration, on the other hand, gas is more evenly distributed between apical and basal regions in normal lungs.[12-14]

With low inspiratory flow rates the distribution of gas depends largely on regional lung compliances, whereas with high flow rates the distribution is dominated by regional resistances. Thus the more compliant basal lung regions receive a greater portion of a slow breath. The resistances in these basal dependent areas are roughly equal to or slightly more than resistances in apical areas. Thus the gas distribution with high inspiratory flow is likewise more equal. As this ventilation becomes more uniform throughout the lung, ventilation-perfusion imbalance could worsen. Indeed, studies in subjects with normal lungs have purported to demonstrate impairment of gas exchange as evidenced by an increased physiologic dead space during mechanical ventilation with increased $\dot{V}I$.[15,16] The changes, however, were inconsistent and too small to be of any clinical significance.

Data obtained with mechanical lung models[17] also suggest that with parallel lung compartments possessing different time constants due either to differences in regional compliance or resistance, the distribution of ventilation between the two areas should become more and more uneven as flow rates increase. Based on such modeling systems, a strong consensus has developed to provide mechanical ventilation with low $\dot{V}I$ rates and hence prolonged TI in most patients with chronic airway obstruction.

Such patients with chronic bronchitis appear to have a normal distribution of airway resistance but a reduced compliance in the dependent lung zones. They therefore exhibit a much reduced basal ventilation compared to normals when inspiratory flow rates are low.[18] With a fast inspiration the distribution of ventilation becomes more normal; i.e., basal areas now receive more ventilation. Connors et al.[19] demonstrated that patients with severe chronic airway obstruction who received mechanical ventilation for respiratory failure had improved gas exchange as V̇I was increased. There was a significant improvement in lung compliance, arterial oxygenation, and physiologic dead space as V̇I was increased from 40 to 100 liters/min. The high V̇I also allows for shorter TI and thus more time for expiration and complete emptying of obstructed airways.[20] These are critical factors in reducing pulmonary hyperinflation and its attendant circulatory depression and barotrauma. In patients with respiratory failure without chronic airways obstruction, the prolonged expiratory time is not as important. Hence the effects of increased V̇I are not as dramatic.[19]

Fresh Gas Flow Rates. The VT delivered by a mechanical ventilator, in particular anesthesia ventilators, is affected by the fresh gas flow (FGF) into the circuit.[11] This is because during inspiration the gas delivered to the lungs comes not only from that in the ventilator bellows but also from the FGF. The latter is continuous throughout the respiratory cycle and not vented during inspiration. Thus the augmentation of VT by FGF is a function of the latter's magnitude and the duration of inspiration (TI), i.e., $\Delta V_T = (FGF \times T_I)$. As respiratory rate (f) decreases, TI becomes longer as a fixed component of each breath. Also, as the ratio of TI to expiratory time increases, TI becomes longer at any given rate. In either case the effects of FGF on VT are increased.[21]

The absolute magnitude of VT augmentation is independent of VT. Thus the percent increase in VT is far greater at the lower VT settings in pediatric patients and may result in considerable hyperventilation and high airway pressures. In practice, however, the augmentation of VT is offset somewhat by the high airway pressures interacting with circuit distensibility and the effects of gas compression.[22]

End-Inspiratory Pause. The end-inspiratory pause is a maneuver that may occur as part of the inspiratory cycle. This represents a period of zero flow that is accomplished by preventing the expiratory valve from opening for a short time after the VT has been delivered and gas flow has ceased. During this period while the lungs are held inflated, the dynamic peak pressure in the circuit decreases to a lower plateau pressure (see Fig. 1.5). Since this plateau pressure more truly reflects the distending pressure in the alveoli of the ventilated lung, it can be used to estimate static lung compliance. More important, the end-inspiratory pause appears to improve gas distribution throughout various areas of the lung and thus improves ventilation-perfusion matching.[23] It is important to note that the use of the inspiratory pause increases TI and consequently P̄aw is also increased accordingly.

Peak Inspiratory Pressure. The maximum airway pressure developed during a mechanically delivered inspiration is referred to as the peak inspiratory or peak inflation pressure. This pressure results from the elastic and flow-resistive properties of the lungs and chest wall and the dynamics of the entire ventilator circuit, including the endotracheal tube. The magnitude of this peak pressure is related to the entire ventilator circuit, including the endotracheal tube. The magnitude of this peak pressure is related to four basic factors (Fig. 9.5). These include delivered volume (VT), inspiratory flow (V̇I), dynamic respiratory compliance, and airway resistance. Increasing levels of VT are associated with higher peak pressures (Fig. 9.5**A**), as are higher V̇I values (Fig. 9.5**B**). The latter can deliver the desired VT in a shorter time and thus a lower $\overline{P}$aw results. Nevertheless, more pressure is lost to the patient circuit and airway resistance. When other variables remain constant, any increase in resistance results in a proportional increase in pressure (Fig. 9.5**C**). Finally, the slope of the pressure curve and peak pressure are inversely related to compliance (Fig. 9.5**D**). An awareness of all of the variables and their interrelationships is essential for understanding the mechanics of ventilatory support.

Termination of Inspiration

The termination of the inspiratory cycle or the change from inspiration to expiration during mechanical ventilation is usually termed cycling. Such cycling can be performed by time, volume, pressure, and sometimes flow. The term "limit" is also applied to the process but indicates that some parameter (usually pressure or volume) is set for a maximum allowable value. An example of such a limit is the pressure relief valve on most anesthesia ventilators, which can be set to vent off excess gases when a certain selected pressure is reached. The latter pressure, however, does not result in actually terminating inspiration. Rather, pressure is held constant and volume delivery ceases until the cycle is completed.

Expiratory Phase

Normal exhalation is a passive process caused by lung and chest wall recoil. The flow is determined by the pressure gradient between the airways and the atmo-

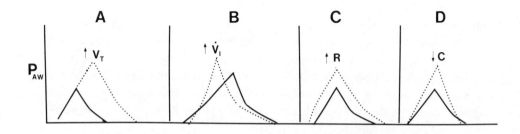

Figure 9.5. Normal pressure-time curves for four inspiratory cycles *(solid lines)* are plotted with the changes *(dotted lines)* produced by (**A**) increased tidal volume (VT), (**B**) increased inspiratory flow (V̇I), (**C**) increased resistance (R), and (**D**) decreased compliance (C). *Paw*, pressure in proximal airway.

sphere. This is offset by resistance to flow provided by the airways, tubing, and valves in the ventilator circuit. The phase of expiration can be altered by expiratory resistance (retard) and the application of negative or positive end-expiratory pressures. Normally, however, the duration of expiratory flow is brief. The total expiratory time (TE) includes not only the period of expiratory flow but also the interval between cessation of flow and initiation of a subsequent inspiration. Typically with normal spontaneous respiration the inspiratory time (TI) constitutes 30 to 40% of the total respiratory cycle (TT) with TE making up the remaining 60 to 70%. The duration of inspiration in relation to that of expiration is termed the I:E ratio. Thus, normal I:E ratios with spontaneous ventilation are about 1:2. With mechanical ventilation, increased I:E ratios (i.e., 1:1 or 2:1 and higher) are usually associated with significantly increased $\overline{Paw}$ and adverse hemodynamic consequences. Values smaller than 1:2 (i.e., 1:3, 1:4, etc.) are associated with lower $\overline{Paw}$ and allow for better alveolar emptying. However, very low I:E ratios (e.g., 1:6), while they decrease $\overline{Paw}$, allow too little time for inspiration and may impair gas exchange accordingly.

The I:E ratio, although popular, does not provide a true perspective of the relationships of TI and TE to total respiratory cycle time (TT) and respiratory rates (f). To determine f, for example, one must first add I + E to determine TT and then see how many cycles occur in 1 minute or, more appropriately, 60 seconds (f = 60T). Physiologists prefer to use the relationships of TI/TT to characterize I:E relationships rather than I:E ratios. Comparative values of TI/TT and I:E are listed in Table 9.1. Note, for example, that an I:E ratio of 1:2 corresponds to a TI/TT of 0.33, or ⅓ the total cycle time.

Auto PEEP and Hyperinflation. The lung volume at the end of exhalation (VEE) in normal adults results from a balance of elastic force of the chest wall acting outward against the inward recoil of the lung. When exhalation ceases, alveolar pressure is usually zero (atmospheric). Normally this occurs at the static resting or relaxation volume of the respiratory system (VRX), which is used interchangeably with functional residual capacity (see Chapter 1). In patients with obstructed airways the time required for exhalation is increased, and VEE is often higher than VRX because dynamic airway collapse and flow

Table 9.1.
Comparison of Inspiratory Duty Cycle (TI/TT) and I:E Ratios

TI/TT	I:E Ratio
0.20	1:4
0.25	1:3
0.33	1:2
0.40	1:1.5
0.50	1:1
0.67	2.1
0.80	4.1

limitation cause "air trapping." The elevation of V$_{EE}$ above V$_{RX}$ is referred to as dynamic hyperinflation.

Dynamic hyperinflation has also been noted in patients during mechanical ventilation for acute exacerbations of respiratory failure. With such air trapping alveolar pressure may not decrease to zero at the end of exhalation. This phenomenon has been referred to as "auto PEEP,"[24] but other terms such as "inadvertent PEEP" have also been used. The auto PEEP usually results from an expiratory time that is too short. Thus air trapping occurs and alveolar pressure remains increased at V$_{EE}$.

The pressure increase may be dangerous because it is not reflected in the usual measurements of proximal airway pressure unless the expiration port on the ventilator circuit is occluded immediately prior to inspiration. The presence of auto PEEP and hyperinflation can be identified by simply disconnecting the ventilator at end exhalation and observing whether the V$_{EE}$ decreases (Fig. 9.6). The amount of volume exhaled during apnea corresponds to the volume of gas "trapped," or the amount of hyperinflation.

Patients with obstructive airway disease may develop significant hyperinflation when ventilatory requirements are high and airflow obstruction is severe. This hyperinflation is associated with an increased risk of barotrauma and circulatory depression. The prime determinants of such hyperinflation are the delivered volume (V$_T$), the expiratory time (T$_E$), and the severity of obstruction. Tuxen et al.[20] have shown that the ventilatory patterns that minimized hyperinflation used increased T$_E$ or decreased V$_T$. The T$_E$ was best increased by reducing f and delivering V$_T$ at an increased $\dot{V}_I$.

Prior recommendations for reduced $\dot{V}_I$ in patients with airflow obstruction were based on concerns about the distribution of ventilation and even more about high peak inspiratory pressures. However, Tuxen et al.[20] suggest that a large component of this peak pressure is dissipated by the airways and endotracheal tube to overcome the high resistance. The peak pressure did not appear to reflect alveolar pressure, the degree of hyperinflation, or circulatory depression. Thus the increased $\dot{V}_I$ may have a beneficial effect largely by deliv-

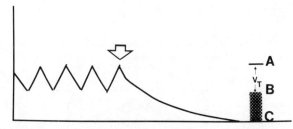

Figure 9.6. Schematic representation of the difference in end-expiratory volume during mechanical ventilation and with a period of apnea begun at *arrow*. *A,* volume at end inspiration after delivery of tidal volume; *B,* end-expiratory volume with ventilation; *C,* end-expiratory volume during apnea, true functional residual capacity. The *shaded portion* represents the gas "trapped" during ventilation.

ering VT quickly so as to allow a greater time for expiration and more complete lung emptying.

Termination of Expiration

The termination of the expiratory phase is accomplished by initiating an inspiration. Like the termination of inspiration, this cycling may occur with time or pressure. Volume and flow mechanisms are theoretically possible but seldom used. A more useful classification categorizes the cycling as controlled or assisted ventilation. With controlled ventilation the expiratory phase is time cycled such that changeover from expiration to inspiration occurs with a timing mechanism that is set and not subject to any outside influence. This initiation of inspiration occurs automatically and is completely independent of patient effort. A similar cycling mechanism for the ventilator occurs during intermittent mandatory ventilation (IMV). With assisted ventilation, pressure cycling is used to initiate inspiration. When the pressure in the upper airway reaches a predetermined value below ambient pressure, the ventilator cycles into inspiration and begins to deliver a breath. If this pressure is a very low value, the ventilator sensitivity to cycling is said to be increased, that is to say, less patient effort will be required to trigger inspiration. The pressure cycling with assisted ventilation is usually superseded by a time-cycling mechanism if a pressure is not generated within a preset time.

REFERENCES

1. Boros SW, Matalon SV, Ewald R, Leonard AS, Hunt CF. The effect of independent variations in inspiratory-expiratory ratio and end expiratory pressure during mechanical ventilation in hyaline membrane disease: the significances of mean airway pressure. J Pediatr 1977;91:794–798.
2. Boros SJ. Variations in inspiratory: expiratory ratio and airway pressure wave form during mechanical ventilation: the significance of mean airway pressure. J Pediatr 1979;94:114–117.
3. Kacmarek RM, Dimas S, Reynolds J, Shapiro BA. Technical aspects of positive end-expiratory pressure (PEEP): Part I: physics of PEEP devices. Respir Care 1982;27:1478–1489.
4. Lyon J, Banner MJ; Jaeger MJ, Peterson CV, Gallagher TJ, Modell HJ. Continuous positive airway pressure and expiratory positive airway pressure increase functional residual capacity equivalently. Chest 1986;89:517–521.
5. Hopewell PC. Failure of positive end-expiratory pressure to decrease lung/water content in alloxan-induced pulmonary edema. Am Rev Respir Dis 1979;120:813–819.
6. Vanderzee H, Cooper JA, Hakin TS, Malik AB. Alterations in pulmonary fluid balance induced by positive end-expiratory pressures. Respir Physiol 1986;64:125–133.
7. Pare PD, Warriner B, Baille EM, Hogg JC. Redistribution of pulmonary extravascular water with positive end-expiratory pressure in canine pulmonary edema. Am Rev Respir Dis 1986;127:590–593.
8. Cassidy SS, Eshenbacher WL, Robertson CH, et al. Cardiovascular effects of positive pressure ventilation in normal subjects. J Appl Physiol 1979;47:453–461.
9. Butler J, Culver BH, Huscby H, Silbert R. The hemodynamics of pulmonary edema. Am Rev Respir Dis 1977;115:173–180.
10. Durinsky PM, Whitcomb ME. The effect of PEEP on cardiac output. Chest 1980;84:210–216.
11. Mushin MW, Rendell-Baker L, Thompson PW, Mapleson WW. Automatic ventilation of the lungs. 3rd ed. Oxford, England: Blackwell, 1980:132–151.

12. Marks JD, Schapera A, Kraemer RW, Katz JA. Pressure and flow limitations of anesthesia ventilators. Anesthesiology 1989;71:403–408.
13. Robertson PC, Anthonisen NR, Ross D. Effect of inspiratory flow rate on regional distribution of inspired gas. J Appl Physiol 1969;26:438–443.
14. Bake B, Wood L, Murphy B, Macklem P, Millic-Emili J. Effect of inspiratory flow rate on regional distribution of inspired gas. J Appl Physiol 1974;38:8–17.
15. Fairley HB, Blenkarn GD. Effect on pulmonary gas exchange of variations in inspiratory flow rate during intermittent positive pressure ventilation. Br J Anaesth 1966;38:320–328.
16. Sykes MK, Lumley J. The effect of varying inspiratory: expiratory ratios on gas exchange during anesthesia for open heart surgery. Br J Anaesth 1969;41:374–380.
17. Jansson L, Johnson B. A theoretical study on flow patterns of ventilators. Scand J Respir Dis 1972;53:237–246.
18. Hughes JMB, Grant BJB, Greene RE, Iliff LD, Milic-Emili J. Inspiratory flow rate and ventilation distribution in normal subjects and in patients with chronic bronchitis. Clin Sci 1972;43:583–595.
19. Connors AF, McCaffree DR, Gray B. Effect of inspiratory flow rate on gas exchange during mechanical ventilation. Am Rev Respir Dis 1981;124:537–543.
20. Tuxen DV, Lane S. The effects of ventilatory pattern on hyperinflation, airway pressures, and circulation in mechanical ventilation of patients with severe airflow obstruction. Am Rev Respir Dis 1987;136:872–879.
21. Gravenstein N, Banner MJ, McLaughlin G. Tidal volume changes due to the interaction of anesthesia machine and ventilator. J Clin Monit 1987;3:187–190.
22. Cote CJ, Petkau AJ, Ryan JF, Welch JP. Wasted ventilation measures in vitro with eight anesthetic circuits with and without incline humidification. Anesthesiology 1983;59:442–446.
23. Fuleihan SF, Wilson RS, Pontoppidan H. Effect of mechanical ventilation with end-inspiratory pause on blood gas exchange. Anesth Analg 1976;55:122–130.
24. Pepe PE, Marcini JJ. Occult positive and expiratory pressure in mechanically ventilated patients with airflow obstruction. Am Rev Respir Dis 1982;126:166–170.

Chapter 10

Monitoring Respiratory Mechanics during Mechanical Ventilation

Monitoring techniques during mechanical ventilation are directed at either the respiratory outcome as reflected by gas exchange or the mechanical demands of the respiratory system. The latter includes both the load imposed by the respiratory system and the patient's ability to handle the load. In ambulatory patients such factors can be evaluated by pulmonary function testing. Unfortunately, the voluntary effort and cooperation required for such testing are seldom possible in patients receiving mechanical ventilation. This chapter focuses on techniques for assessing the physical properties of the lungs and chest wall. The initial discussion centers on the primary measurements of pressure, volume, and flow. This is followed by a discussion of the application of these primary measurements to assessing mechanical demand and capability, including approaches to weaning from mechanical ventilation.

AIRWAY PRESSURE

The distention and collapse of the lungs during mechanical ventilation are governed by the same pressure gradients as during spontaneous ventilation. However, the respiratory cycles differ somewhat. For example, with spontaneous ventilation pressure and flow vary in rather sinusoidal fashion with time, whereas with mechanical ventilation the flow pattern is usually more constant and the inspiratory pressure trace terminates abruptly. The mechanically delivered breaths also tend to be associated with a higher mean airway pressure, which may have adverse cardiovascular effects.

Of greatest interest to the clinical physiologist would be a direct measurement of the pressure within the airway, in particular the trachea. Since this is not usually accessible, pressure in the external airway (Paw), or more specifically airways opening, is usually measured with a needle manometer or pressure transducer connected to a tap that enters the airway at a 90° angle. The

167

transducer is desirable since it provides the opportunity for a graphic display of pressure over the time of a respiratory cycle.

During a mechanical inflation the maximal or peak airway pressure (Ppk) indicates the dynamic pressure (Fig. 10.1) that results from attempting to distend the respiratory system with a given tidal volume (V_T) delivered at a given inspiratory flow ($\dot{V}_I$). Absolute values for Ppk depend on the impedance of the respiratory system, the ventilator settings (V_T and $\dot{V}_I$) and the resistance of the apparatus between the sampling site and lungs. The principal resistance is that of the endotracheal tube, whose narrow channel can be further compromised by kinks, secretions, or impingement of the tip against the airway wall. These will serve to elevate Ppk, whereas a cuff leak may decrease it. If V_T and $\dot{V}_I$ flow patterns remain the same, Ppk measurements may be useful to identify such changes and may also reflect bronchoconstriction or dilation.

When the airway is occluded at end inspiration and flow ceases ($\dot{V}_I = 0$), the Ppk delays rapidly to a plateau value at end inspiration (PEI). As gas distribution equalizes throughout the lungs, the speed of this equilibration depends on the homogeneity of regional time constants. Regions with high alveolar pressure and volume tend to empty into undistended areas with low pressure and prolonged time constants. This process is abnormally prolonged in patients with chronic obstructive pulmonary disease.

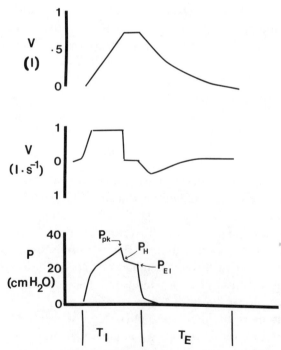

Figure 10.1. Flow (liters/sec), pressure (cm H_2O), and volume (liters) during mechanical ventilation incorporating an inspiratory pause. Ppk, peak inspiratory pressure; PH pressure at the beginning of the hold or pause; PEI plateau pressure at end inspiration.

Usually PEI values are several centimeters of H_2O less than pressures recorded at the instant flow ceases (PH) and the inspiratory hold or pause begins (Fig. 10.1). The inability to develop a stable PEI may indicate a leak in the circuit and would be an expected observation in the presence of a bronchopulmonary fistula. At zero flow during end inspiration, PEI measured in the proximal airways reflects alveolar pressure well and can be used to characterize the elastic recoil of the respiratory system, provided a sufficient pause time is possible. As a quasistatic measurement, PEI is not affected by secretions, bronchospasm, or any other forms of airways obstruction.

PLEURAL PRESSURE

In the clinical setting direct measurement of pleural pressure (Ppl) is seldom used, largely because of difficulty in estimating Ppl. Within the thorax Ppl varies from site to site because of lung geometry and hydrostatic forces. In the apical or nondependent areas Ppl is more negative than at the basal or dependent lung regions. The variation in Ppl is about 0.25 cm H_2O for each centimeter of lung vertical distance, largely the result of hydrostatic forces.

Estimation of Ppl is helpful in separating the mechanical properties of the lungs and chest wall. Lung inflation during spontaneous or mechanical ventilation is accomplished by changes in transpulmonary pressure (PL), which is the difference between airway pressure (Paw)—or more specifically, alveolar pressure (PA)—and Ppl. The inspiratory expansion of the chest wall is reflected by changes in Ppl relative to atmospheric pressure.

To estimate Ppl a balloon-catheter system is usually introduced into the lower esophagus.[1] The balloon is usually 10 cm in length and thus able to sense local pleural pressure over a sizable segment of esophageal length. The balloon reflects changes in Ppl and esophageal pressure (Pes) acceptably, provided esophageal muscle contraction does not occur. A number of techniques have been described for determining balloon placement, usually by measuring pressure swings during forced inhalation maneuvers.[1,2] Clinical measurement of Pes has been aided by the development of a nasogastric esophageal balloon system.[3] The balloon in this system is incorporated into a standard nasogastric tube. This appears to be ideally suited for patients receiving mechanical ventilation, since many require nasogastric tube placement. Comparison with the standard intraesophageal balloon measurements suggest that the nasogastric system provides acceptable measurement of Pes for studying lung and chest wall mechanics.[4]

FLOW

The measurement of airflow during mechanical ventilation is essential for estimating resistance, since the latter is the ratio of the driving pressure between the airway opening and alveoli and flow. In the clinical setting the flow tracing can also be utilized for purposes other than the estimation of resistance. For example, ripples on the inspiratory waveform suggest turbulent flow and the high likelihood of airway secretions. Expiratory flow normally decays in an exponential fashion, so if the decay profile is linear, expiratory flow limitation is likely. Furthermore, if flow persists at the end of exhalation (i.e., the beginning of the subsequent inspiration), hyperinflation is likely since the resting equilibrium position of the respiratory system is not reached.

Techniques for measuring flow can be functionally divided into those that use pressure gradient–based devices and those that use non–pressure-based devices. Of the pressure-based devices available to measure flow, the pneumotachograph is perhaps the best known.[5] A low mechanical resistance, usually in the form of capillary tubes or a screen, is placed directly in the stream of gas flow. The pressure gradient across this resistance is sensed by a differential pressure transducer and is linearly related to flow if flow is laminar. To ensure such linearity, it is important to select the pneumotachograph that is linear in the flow rates likely to be experienced (e.g., for forced expiration, 6 to 10 liters/sec; for quiet tidal volume, 0 to 1 liter/sec).

The pressure gradient is dependent not only on the flow rate but also on the density and viscosity of the gas mixture as well as its temperature. Furthermore, condensation of moisture may increase screen resistance and cause turbulence. The latter is usually eliminated by electrically heating the screen. Despite these limitations, the rapid response, small dead space, and low resistance of the pneumotachograph render it useful for flow measurement in many situations. Also, when this flow is integrated electronically with respect to time, a measurement of volume can be derived.

The non–pressure-based devices for flow measurement include hot wire spirometers, ultrasonic flow meters, and vortex shedding pneumotachographs. With the thermal-based or hot wire spirometer, a heated wire or thermistor is cooled by the gas stream to an extent related to flow rate and thermal conductivity of the gas. Thus the amount of additional current required to maintain the temperature of the wire is related to flow. Such thermally based devices are robust and easily sterilized and are suitable for applications not requiring a high degree of accuracy. They diminish in sensitivity rapidly if coated with foreign debris such as airway secretions.

The velocity of gas flow can also be measured by utilizing ultrasound. The basis for ultrasonic flowmeters is the measurement of the change in the speed of sound. Two piezoelectric crystals aligned at angles to the gas flow alternately transmit and receive bursts of oscillations at a frequency of 100 kHz. Such flowmeters have advantages over pneumotachographs in certain situations because of their low resistance. They also do not have problems with moisture, positive pressure, or motion artifact, and they tend to be more stable; i.e., they exhibit less drift over long periods of use.

Vortex shedding pneumotachographs utilize obstructing struts placed in the airstream to disrupt laminar flow.[5] When the smoothly moving air encounters such obstructions, turbulence results. The degree of turbulence generated is directly related to the speed of airflow. Each individual turbulent swirl is referred to as a vortex. Downstream of the strut a sensor detects an ultrasonic beam projected across the tube. The vortices interrupt the beam and generate a pulse with each deflection. The electrical pulses are counted and correlated to flow. Such devices have minimal dead space and are insensitive to gas composition. Their major problem lies in the design, which limits sensitivity to either high or low flow ranges. Because they rely on the creation of turbulence, very low flows may not disrupt the laminar flow sufficiently to produce turbulence. Conversely, if the device is designed to measure slow flow, rapid airflow may produce such excessive turbulence that vortices cannot be counted. Another problem quite relevant to mechanically ventilated patients relates to the influence of water condensation. Although not highly affected by humidity, vortex pneumotachographs may give erroneous values if water condenses on struts or sensors.

VOLUME

Volumes delivered during mechanical ventilation can be measured accurately by electronic integration of the measured airflow signal provided by a pneumotachograph. Other determination of delivered volume can be provided by collection devices such as dry gas meters, mechanical spirometers, or respirometers, and devices that track thoracoabdominal movement.

Dry gas meters (Parkinson-Cowan) have been used to measure minute ventilation for extended periods. The gas meters have too large an internal volume and a large amount of dead space to allow rebreathing. Rather, gas must be collected via a one-way valve on the expiratory limb or in a Douglas bag, which is then emptied into the meters. The gas volumes are collected at ambient temperature and pressure saturated with H_2O vapor (ATPS), but for precision, respiratory volumes are expressed at body temperature and pressure saturated with H_2O vapor (BTPS). Many tables are available for such conversion factors, which are calculated as follows:

$$\text{BTPS vol} = \text{ATPS vol} \times \frac{(273 \times \text{Tb}^\circ\text{C})}{(273 \times \text{Tatm}^\circ\text{C})} \times \frac{(\text{Patm} - \text{P}_{H_2O}\ \text{Tb})}{(\text{Patm} - \text{P}_{H_2O}\ \text{Tatm})}$$

where Tb is body temperature, Tatm is atmospheric temperature, P_{H_2O} is vapor pressure of H_2O at Tb or Tatm, and Patm is atmospheric or barometric pressure.

The classic Collins water seal spirometers are reliable and accurate, and they serve as the reference standard for volume measurements. However, they are cumbersome and poorly suited for use in the operating room or intensive care unit. Dry spirometers, such as the rolling seal or wedge types, have similar problems of bulk but have better frequency response, which renders them more useful for forced respiratory maneuvers. In addition, they often have electrical circuitry capable of differentiating the volume signal to obtain flow. The principal shortcoming of such spirometers lies in the difficulty of applying them to systems in which rebreathing takes place or additional fresh gas is added to the volume inspired.

In contrast to the limitations of conventional spirometers, mechanical respirometers provide a less expensive, more convenient access to the breathing circuit. Such devices estimate volume from the rotation of a low-friction inertia vane. The widely used Wright respirometer contains a geared system that converts rotation of the vane into movements of hands on a dial. Tangential slots around the vane ensure that flow is recorded in only one direction. Thus, the vane may be inserted between the endotracheal tube and the breathing circuit. The small dead space (20 to 25 ml) and relatively low resistance render it suitable for patients who are breathing spontaneously. The instrument is more accurate at flows of about 20 liters/min. These flows are typical of quiet expiration in adults. Because of the inertia, resistance, and momentum of the vane, the Wright respirometer tends to overread at higher flows and underread at lower flows. Although changes in gas composition have relatively little effect, water condensation is often a problem after extended use, as is accumulation of foreign material.

These problems of the Wright respirometer are shared by a number of similar devices. Such is the case with the larger, widely used Drager respirometer. This equipment senses flow in either direction and must, of necessity, be placed in an area of undirectional flow on the expiratory limb of an anesthesia circuit system. Such placement of the respirometer renders it prone to overreading, because of increases in fresh gas delivery to the system, particularly when such delivered flows are large (e.g., 10 liters/min).

Konno and Mead[6] have measured movements of the chest wall and abdomen and demonstrated their relationships to tidal volume during unobstructed respiration. Various transducers and devices have measured the changes in physical shape and hence the electrical properties of the chest and abdomen during respiration.[7] These devices have consisted of mercury in rubber strain gauges, magnetometers, impedance electrodes, and, most recently, the inductance plethysmograph (Respitrace, Ambulatory Monitoring, Ardsley, NY). This device consists of two insulated coils, one of which encircles the abdomen and the other the rib cage. The coils are contained within a netlike garment and are excited by a high-frequency oscillation. The inductance of the coils changes with respiration as a function of changes in the cross-sectional area of the compartment enclosed within. The instrument is useful for detecting apnea and eliminates the need for mouthpieces or masks. For measurement of volumes, however, devices such as the Respitrace must be regarded as semiquantitative, unless rigorous calibrations with a spirometer are repeatedly carried out.

TIDAL VOLUME: DELIVERED VERSUS EXHALED

During mechanical ventilation the tidal volume delivered by the ventilator and the volume exhaled usually differ. Of the possible causes of this difference a circuit leak is quite common and is easily detected and corrected. Another major cause of the difference is the fresh gas flow. The impact of the latter is greatest with high fresh gas flows and prolonged inspiratory times (see Chapter 9).

Tidal volumes measured during mechanical ventilation also differ from those actually reaching the patient because a certain portion of the volume is compressed within the ventilator and circuit. This is referred to as the compression volume and helps to explain the high volumes required during mechanical ventilation compared to spontaneous breathing. As pressure rises within the circuit, the tubing also elongates and distends. During exhalation this gas volume is released without having entered the lung. These volumes are of great importance in infants but may also be significant in adult patients who require high inflation pressures because of increased airway resistance or decreased compliance.

The compression volume is in a sense apparatus dead space or a form of wasted ventilation. An estimation of its magnitude necessitates considering Ppk and the total circuit volume exclusive of the lung. Boyle's law can then be used to calculate compression volume. For example, if peak airway pressure is 40 mm Hg (about 54 cm H_2O) and the circuit volume (V_1) is 10 liters, the volume of the circuit during compression (V_2) can be calculated using atmospheric pressure (P_1) as 760 and the absolute ventilatory pressure (P_2) as $P_1 + 40 = 800$.

$$P_1V_1 = P_2V_2$$
$$760 \times 10 \text{ liters} = 800 \times V_2$$
$$V_2 = 9.5 \text{ liters}$$

Thus 0.5 liter of gas has been compressed in the circuit without ever reaching the lung. If a spirometer is mounted in the circuit just before the expiratory valve, a measured tidal volume of 1.0 liter would include about 50 ml of the compression volume. Exhaled volume must be measured mouthward from the circuit Y-piece (i.e., at the endotracheal tube) to avoid this error in estimating tidal volume.

MONITORING MECHANICAL DEMAND

Compliance

Conventionally, compliance (i.e., the static volume-pressure relationship) of the respiratory system has been assessed in ventilated patients with the super syringe method.[8] This consists of inflating the relaxed respiratory system to several volumes above FRC within the patient's range of tidal volume (up to 1.5 liters). Each step is held for several seconds until a plateau pressure is maintained. The technique requires disconnection of the patient from the ventilator and may therefore present a hazard. Furthermore, the measurements are based on the assumption that the thoracic volume and syringe volume are equal. However, with time there is a fall in thoracic volume in paralyzed subjects due to continuing gas exchange.[9] The latter may result in a decreased value for compliance measured during deflation unless the inflation-deflation sequence is accomplished rapidly.

During delivery of the tidal volume from a ventilator, airway pressure rises to a peak at end inspiration and is then followed by a rapid fall to base line during expiration. The peak pressure (Ppk) reflects the forces required to overcome the elastic recoil of the respiratory system and the frictional resistance of the airways. If the delivered tidal volume (VT) is divided by Ppk the value is often referred to as the dynamic compliance (Cdyn). This terminology has been criticized because Cdyn actually represents more of an impedance measurement that includes compliance and resistance components. The term "dynamic characteristic" has been proposed as an index of this overall difficulty of expanding the respiratory system.[10]

Determination of the static compliance (Cst) of the respiratory system is aided by the built-in devices in modern ventilators that allow an end-inspiratory occlusion or pause. If occlusion is held until a plateau end-inspiratory pressure (PEI) is reached (Fig. 10.1), Cst can then be estimated by dividing the delivered VT by PEI.

Another useful form of quasi-static compliance measurement applicable to ventilator patients receiving constant inspiratory flow is a pulse method, which quantitates pressure rise per unit time during such flow.[11] It is based on the principle that when a constant flow is introduced to the respiratory system, the rate of increase in pressure is inversely related to the compliance of the system (Fig. 10.2).[12]

$$\text{Compliance} = \frac{\text{flow}}{\Delta \text{ pressure/time}}$$

Since flow $= \Delta \text{ volume/time}$,

$$\text{Compliance} = \frac{\Delta \text{ volume}}{\Delta \text{ pressure}}$$

Values for compliance estimated by this method should be nearly identical to those obtained by relating delivered VT to the plateau pressure (PEI) and are therefore also considered quasi-static. The measurement of compliance with this pulse method reflects the true static compliance both in normal subjects[13]

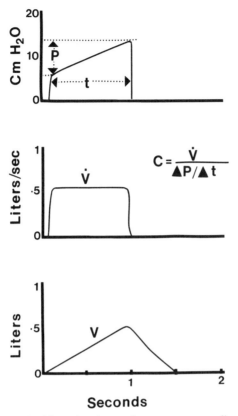

Figure 10.2. The pulse method for estimating respiratory system compliance (C) by dividing constant inspiratory flow ($\dot{V}$) by the rate of pressure rise ($\triangle P/\triangle T$). (Reproduced with permission from Gal TJ. Monitoring the function of the respiratory system. In: Lake CL, ed. Clinical monitoring. Philadelphia: WB Saunders, 1989:321–332.)

and in patients with abnormal lung mechanics and inhomogeneity of gas mixing within the lungs.[11]

Resistance

When the respiratory system is inflated with a constant flow, a characteristic airway pressure pattern occurs from which some estimates of respiratory system mechanics can be obtained. The initial change in pressure (Fig. 10.3) indicates pressure loss (Pr) across resistive elements that must be overcome before a volume change can occur. In ventilated patients Pr reflects the resistance of the endotracheal tube and airways, with some minor contribution from the viscous resistance of the lung and chest wall as well as respiratory system inertance. During ventilation with such a "square-wave" flow, inspiratory resistance can theoretically be calculated by dividing Pr by the inspiratory flow. Estimation of Pr requires extrapolating the airway pressure ramp back to the time at which flow begins (Fig. 10.3).[14] The increase of Pr above baseline end-expira-

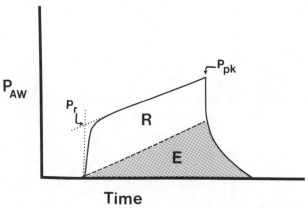

Figure 10.3.   Airway pressure trace during inflation at a constant inspiratory flow. The *shaded area* (E) reflects the pressure to overcome elastic forces. Area R reflects the resistive or frictional forces required for flow. Pr, approximation of pressure at the onset of inspiration estimated by extrapolating back to time zero on the pressure trace.

tory pressure reflects the pressure gradient between the airway opening and alveoli before any alteration in elastic forces associated with volume change occurs. Unfortunately, this technique may yield inaccuracies if the airway pressure is not truly linear, if hyperinflation or "auto PEEP" is present, or if resistance is volume dependent; i.e., the pressure gradient between airway opening and alveoli is greater at the onset compared to the termination of inflation.

After the initial pressure change (Pr) at the onset of inflation, airway pressure increases in linear fashion to a maximal or peak (Ppk) value (Fig. 10.1). The slope of the pressure trace is related to the inspiratory flow rate and even more importantly to the elastic properties of the respiratory system. As mentioned previously, the latter serves as the basis for the pulse method of calculating compliance. The maximal pressure at end inspiration (Ppk) is the total dynamic pressure required for delivery of the set volume at the set flow. The Ppk reflects both resistive and elastic forces. If a pause is introduced at end inspiration, Ppk decreases to P$_{EI}$ (Fig. 10.1), which reflects primarily the elastic forces. The total effective or maximal resistance at end inspiration (Rmax) can thus be calculated by dividing the difference between peak dynamic pressure (Ppk) and static airway pressure (P$_{EI}$) by the delivered flow at the moment of Ppk.[15] This Rmax consists of the intrinisic or pure flow resistance (Rmin) and an effective additional resistance ($\triangle$R), which reflects inequalities in the regional time constants.[15] Calculation of Rmin utilizes the difference between Ppk and the pressure at the onset of the inspiratory pause or occlusion (P$_H$), while $\triangle$R is estimated from differences between P$_H$ and P$_{EI}$. The accuracy of the latter pressure is highly dependent on a sufficiently long pause to allow pressure to equilibrate in the face of regional lung inhomogeneities. The magnitude of Rmin is highly dependent on inspiratory flow rate (V̇$_I$) and inflation volume.[15] At a given inflation volume, for example, Rmin increases directly with increasing $\dot{V}_I$, because of the marked dropoff from Ppk to P_H at the onset of the inspiratory pause.[15] On the other hand, with a constant $\dot{V}_I$, increasing inflation volume produces a decreased Rmin, although $\triangle R$ increases somewhat.

In many disease states, especially those associated with airway obstruction, the resistance to airflow during exhalation is usually greater than that during inspiration. Calculations of the expiratory resistance can be made from estimates of alveolar pressure (P_A) and flow ($\dot{V}$). The P_A can be estimated by stopping flow during exhalation by occluding the expiratory port for at least 0.5 second.[16] This stop-flow condition allows airway pressure and P_A to equilibrate. Resistance is volume dependent, i.e., it increases as lung volume decreases. Therefore, several such stop-flow measurements may be necessary in patients with obstructive airway disease to characterize the magnitude of resistance over the full range of exhaled volume.

Expiratory resistance can be estimated by using the time constant (τ) of passive exhalation. When one time constant has elapsed since the beginning of exhalation 37% of the delivered volume (V_T) remains in the lungs; i.e., 63% has been exhaled. Since $\tau = R \times C$, the average expiratory resistance can be calculated as $R = \tau/C$, where τ is time in seconds for V_T to decrease to 37% of its end-inspiratory value. The value of C can be computed from the ratio of V_T to P_{EI}.

The estimation of τ can be made from pressure-time curves instead of volume-time curves and may be preferred in the clinical setting. The advantage in using pressure lies in the fact that Paw and hence P_A can be readily obtained by connecting a pressure transducer to the airway. This does not require disconnection from the ventilator or unusually prolonged expiratory times, as might be required to measure exhaled volume accurately in some patients.

WORK OF BREATHING

The work of breathing is essentially the product of the inflating pressure and the delivered volume. This three-dimensional situation in the respiratory system corresponds to the simple physical relationship of force times the distance moved. To measure the mechanical work the product of distending pressure or transpulmonary pressure (P_L) and the rate of volume change is integrated over the duration of a breath. This pressure-volume integral is graphically estimated as the area within a pressure-volume plot (Fig. 10.4).

Under conditions of constant flow, the volume and airway pressure traces are linearly related to time. Thus the airway pressure trace can be used in place of a pressure-volume plot. Both pressure-volume and pressure-time curves (Figs. 10.2 and 10.3) resemble a trapezoid whose area is calculated as the product of the base (time) and the average of the major and minor heights. Thus the pressure at midtidal volume (V_T) provides an estimate of the work required

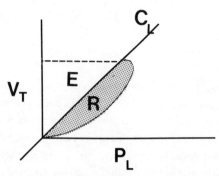

Figure 10.4.   Graphic illustration for the work of inflating the lung with a given tidal volume (V_T). The applied transpulmonary pressure (P_L) works against resistive forces (R) and elastic forces (E). The pressure-volume relationship of the lung, i.e., lung compliance (C_L), is indicated by the slope of the line through points of zero flow.

to inflate the respiratory system to a selected V_T at a given inspiratory flow.[17] An alternative, though not as precise, estimation of the work of breathing can be derived from Ppk and static P_{EI} used for calculations of resistance and compliance. In the paralyzed patient (Ppk − P_{EI})/2 provides an estimate of the work of inflation per liter in cm H_2O, which can be converted to joules by dividing by 10.[17]

DISCONTINUING MECHANICAL VENTILATION

In many patients abrupt termination of mechanical ventilatory support is possible with little or no problem. Others who do not tolerate sudden conversion to spontaneous breathing require a gradual removal of ventilatory support termed "weaning." Difficulty withdrawing ventilatory support in either case usually arises from an imbalance between ventilatory ability and mechanical and metabolic demands. Many clinical criteria have been proposed to monitor breathing effort and predict successful weaning from mechanical ventilation.[18] However, it has been suggested that the physiology of weaning from mechanical ventilation is rather complex and may be more of an art than a science.[19] Furthermore, the actual readiness of the patient is more important for success in discontinuing ventilation than is the method used for weaning.

Ventilatory Demand

The demand for ventilation is a composite of the mechanical work required for gas flow (i.e., the work against elastic and resistive forces) and of the minute ventilation requirement. The latter is determined by three major factors: an increased CO_2 production, impaired ability to excrete CO_2 (wasted ventilation, dead space), and an increased ventilatory response (Table 10.1).

All hypermetabolic states—such as fever, burns, and sepsis—are commonly associated with increased production of CO_2. The output of CO_2 is also significantly increased by the amount and source of calories provided to

Table 10.1.
Factors Increasing Ventilatory Demand

Increased CO_2 Production
Agitation
Fever
Pain
Sepsis
Shivering
High carbohydrate feeding
Increased work of breathing
Increased Dead Space
Obstructive lung disease
Hypovolemia
Decreased cardiac output
Pulmonary emboli
Excessive PEEP
Ventilator circuit
Increased Ventilatory Response
Neurogenic factors
Psychogenic factors (anxiety)
Hypoxemia
Hypotension
Metabolic acidosis

patients. Excessive feeding of carbohydrates may generate more CO_2 than that resulting from fats or protein. Thus ventilatory failure or failure to wean from ventilatory support may result if patients fed excessive carbohydrate loads cannot handle the increased CO_2 production.[20]

Most disease processes that prompt the need for mechanical ventilation significantly affect intrapulmonary gas distribution and thus increase the wasted ventilation or dead space fraction (VD/VT). Other factors not directly related to pathological alterations in lung parenchyma may also increase VD/VT. For example, hypotension or pulmonary emboli may result in decreased pulmonary perfusion, as may the application of excessive levels of PEEP. On the other hand, increased apparatus dead space from the ventilator circuit may also contribute to the VD/VT, especially with the low-volume breaths characteristic of spontaneously breathing patients with respiratory failure.

Ventilatory demand may also increase in the face of an enhanced ventilatory response or central drive to breathe. Central neurogenic hyperventilation may accompany a variety of neurologic disorders. Ventilatory demand may also be accentuated by psychogenic factors such as anxiety and by metabolic factors such as acidosis and hypoxemia. Clinicians should be alerted to the latter factors, since they are reversible with proper treatment.

Ventilatory Performance and Capability

Muscle Strength. Respiratory muscle strength may be assessed by measuring maximum airway pressures (see Chapter 2). The maximum inspiratory pressure (PImax) has become a standard measurement employed to predict the likelihood of discontinuing mechanical ventilation. To measure PImax, inspiratory efforts must begin from a lung volume that ensures the development of maximal force. Although usually measured in the laboratory at residual volume, PImax measurements in the clinical setting are usually made at functional residual capacity, since the measurement then reflects the pressure available for inspiration at the normal end-expiratory lung volume.

As a static (isometric) measurement PImax exceeds maximum pressures achieved under dynamic conditions. As ventilatory requirements and flow rates increase, the disparity between the static PImax and dynamic inspiratory pressures becomes even greater. This is because, as the velocity of muscle contraction increases, the capacity for generating force decreases. A PImax value of at least -30 cm H_2O has been touted as the value at which spontaneous ventilation could be maintained while the patient is extubated.[21] However, other observations indicate that this level of PImax was unreliable as a predictor of success or failure.[22] The modest reliability of PImax perhaps stems from the fact that the measurement does not reflect other important mechanical factors such as respiratory system compliance or resistance. Increases in either of the latter will require a larger fraction of PImax to sustain adequate ventilation.

Vital Capacity.   The size of the vital capacity (VC) provides some information about respiratory muscle strength, but VC is rather disappointing as an actual measure of strength or a predictor of the ability to ventilate. This is largely because the VC is highly subject to patient effort and cooperation as well as lung mechanics. Even in cooperative patients with normal lung mechanics, VC tends to be preserved unless weakness is severe.[23] This results from the curvilinear nature of the pressure-volume curve of the normal respiratory system (see Fig. 1.3). At the extremes of lung volume, large changes in applied pressure are associated with small volume changes. Thus, with large decreases in muscle strength only small decreases in volume occur. Respiratory muscle strength must be decreased by 20% or more before significant reductions in VC occur.

Normal values for VC are about 70 ml/kg. Values greater than 10 ml/kg are regarded as essential for successful cessation of ventilatory support.[24] However, numerous other studies have underscored the poor predictive value of VC, largely because of poor patient cooperation.

Muscle Endurance.   Measurements of ventilatory muscle strength correlate with the ability to sustain ventilation, but the predictive relationships are not as good as measures of endurance. The latter characterize the ability of the respiratory muscles to sustain the load placed on them in the form of both ventilatory demand and mechanics. The relationship between minute ventilation ($\dot{V}E$) and maximum voluntary ventilation (MVV) provides an indication of the reserve energy or potential for endurance. Healthy young subjects can maintain minute ventilations slightly more than half their MVV for extended periods.[25] Conversely, patients who could at least double $\dot{V}E$ voluntarily with an MVV maneuver could undergo successful discontinuance of mechanical ventilation.[20] This suggests that $\dot{V}E/MVV$ ratios of 50% or less reliably indicate that spontaneous ventilation can be adequately maintained.

Such maximum voluntary ventilation efforts require a high degree of patient cooperation and have prompted efforts to estimate endurance with data from spontaneous respiratory cycles devoid of much patient cooperation. The energy required by the inspiratory muscles during contraction is a function of two factors: the force of contraction expressed as a fraction of the maximum capability (PImax) and the duration of contraction, i.e., the inspiratory time fraction (TI/TT). The ratio of the average inspiratory pressure ($\overline{P}I$) to PImax, which relates force of contraction to maximum capability, is usually < 0.4, as is the ratio of TI/TT. The product of the two ratios ($\overline{P}I/PImax \times TI/TT$) has been referred to as the inspiratory effort quotient (IEQ).[19] The calculation has also been termed the "pressure-time index" and correlates well with O_2 consumption.[26] If the IEQ exceeds the critical value of 0.15 to 0.20, the patient is working near the limits of endurance and fatigue is highly likely.

Respiratory Patterns. A very sensitive, though not specific, index of respiratory fatigue is an increase in respiratory frequency. This tachypnea is often accompanied by an uncoordinated pattern of breathing. The high respiratory rates in such patients are hardly optimal because of the increased work of breathing and CO_2 production. Furthermore, the reduced expiratory time may be insufficient for complete emptying of all lung units such that end-expiratory volume increases. This resultant hyperinflation further compromises inspiratory muscle contraction and further increases the work of breathing. The observations of Tobin et al.[27] indicate that failure to ventilate adequately after discontinuance of mechanical ventilation was associated with immediate development of a rapid, shallow breathing pattern. The latter quickly resulted in inefficient gas exchange and hypercapnia.

Ventilatory Drive. One of the requirements for successful spontaneous ventilation is the central ventilatory drive. Many techniques to assess such drive are not practical in critically ill patients. However, occlusion pressure ($P_{0.1}$), the pressure generated in the initial 100 milliseconds following airway occlusion, correlates well with central neural drive in normal subjects[28] and patients.[29] As an isometric measurement $P_{0.1}$ is not affected by respiratory mechanics but is influenced by lung volume and to a mild extent by muscle strength.

During respiratory failure $P_{0.1}$ values are increased[29] and tend to decrease with improving respiratory status. The high $P_{0.1}$ implies an increased respiratory drive, which may lead to inspiratory muscle fatigue. Sassoon et al.[30] found that $P_{0.1}$ was consistently higher in patients who failed to wean from mechanical ventilation. In another study, patients who failed to exhibit measurable increases in $P_{0.1}$ during CO_2 challenge also failed to achieve adequate spontaneous ventilation.[31] These studies provide only limited confirmation of $P_{0.1}$ as a predictor of weaning; however, they do provide some insight as to the role for such indices of ventilatory drive in evaluating the patient receiving mechanical ventilation.

REFERENCES

1. Milic-Emili J, Mead J, Turner JM, et al. Improved techniques for estimating pleural pressure for esophageal balloon. J Appl Physiol 1964;19:207–211.
2. Baydur A, Panagiotis K, Zin WA, Jaeger M, Milic-Emili J. A simple method for assessing the validity of the esophageal balloon technique. Am Rev Respir Dis 1982;126:788–791.
3. Leatherman NE. An improved balloon system for monitoring intraesophageal pressure in acutely ill patients. Crit Care Med 1978;6:189–192.
4. Gillespie DJ. Comparison of intraesophageal balloon pressure measurements with a nasogastric-esophageal balloon system in volunteers. Am Rev Respir Dis 1982;126:583–585.
5. Sullivan W, Peter GM, Enright PL. Pneumotachygraphs: theory and clinical application. Respir Care 1984;29:736–749.
6. Konno K, Mead J. Measurement of the separate volume changes of the rib cage and abdomen during breathing. J Appl Physiol 1967;22:407–422.
7. Cohn MA, Rao ASV, Broudy M, et al. The respiratory inductive plethysmograph: a new noninvasive monitor of respiration. Bull Eur Physiopathol Respir 1982;18:643–658.
8. Bendixen HH, Egbert LD, Hedley White J. Respiratory care. St. Louis: CV Mosby, 1965:50.
9. Dall'ava-Santucci J, Armaganidis A, Brunet F, et al. Causes of error in pressure volume curves in the adult respiratory distress syndrome. J Appl Physiol 1988;64:42–49.
10. Bone RC. Monitoring ventilatory mechanics in acute respiratory failure. Respir Care 1983;28:597–603.
11. Suratt PM, Owens DH. A pulse method of measuring respiratory system compliance in ventilated patients. Chest 1981;80:34–38.
12. Rattenborg CC, Holaday DA. Constant flow inflation of the lungs, theoretical analysis. Acta Anaesthesiol Scand 1967;23:211–223.
13. Suratt PM, Owens DH, Kilgore WT, Harry RR, Hsiao HS. A pulse method of measuring respiratory system compliance. J Appl Physiol 1980;48:1116–1121.
14. Bates JH, Rossi A, Milic-Emili J. Analysis of the behavior of the respiratory system with constant inspiratory flow. J Appl Physiol 1985;58:1840–1848.
15. D'Angelo E, Calderini E, Torri G, Robatto M, Bono D, Milic-Emili J. Respiratory mechanics in anesthetized paralyzed human. Effects of flow, volume, and time. J Appl Physiol 1989;67:2556–2564.
16. Gottfried SB, Rossi A, Higgs BD, et al. Non-invasive determination of respiratory system mechanics during mechanical ventilation for acute respiratory failure. Am Rev Respir Dis 1985;131:414–420.
17. Marinin JJ, Rodriguez RM, Lamb V. Bedside estimation of the inspiratory work of breathing during mechanical ventilation. Chest 1986;89:56–63.
18. Sahn SA, Lakshminarayan S, Petty TL. Weaning from mechanical ventilation. JAMA 1976;235:2208–2212.
19. Milic-Emili J. Is weaning an art or science? Am Rev Respir Dis 1986;134:1108–1110.
20. Covelli HD, Black JW, Olsen MS, Beekmaj JF. Respiratory failure precipitated by high carbohydrate loads. Ann Intern Med 1981;95:579–581.
21. Sahn SA, Lakshminarayan S. Bedside criteria for discontinuation of mechanical ventilation. Chest 1973;63:1002–1005.
22. Tahvainen J, Salenpera M, Nilcki P. Extubation criteria after weaning from intermittent mandatory ventilation and continuous positive airway pressure. Crit Care Med 1983;11:702–707.
23. Gal TJ, Goldberg SK. Relationship between respiratory muscle strength and vital capacity during partial curarization in awake subjects. Anesthesiology 1981;54:141–147.
24. Feeley TW, Hedley-White J. Weaning from mechanical ventilation and supplemental oxygen. N Engl J Med 1975;292:903–906.
25. Zocche GP, Fitts HW, Cournand A. Fraction of maximum breathing capacity available for prolonged hyperventilation. J Appl Physiol 1960;15:1073–1074.
26. Field S, Sanci S, Grassino A. Respiratory muscle oxygen consumption estimated by the diaphragm pressure-time index. J Appl Physiol 1984;57:44–51.
27. Tobin MJ, Perez W, Guenther SM, et al. The pattern of breathing during successful and unsuccessful trials of weaning from mechanical ventilation. Am Rev Respir Dis 1986;134:1111–1118.

28. Whitelaw WA, Derenne JP, Milic-Emili J. Occlusion pressure as a measure of respiratory center output in conscious man. Respir Physiol 1975;23:181–199.
29. Aubier M, Murciano D, Fournier M, Milic-Emili J, Pariente R, Derenne JP. Central respiratory drive in acute respiratory failure of patients with chronic obstructive pulmonary disease. Am Rev Respir Dis 1980;122:191–199.
30. Sassoon CSH, Teresita TT, Mahutte CK, Light RW. Airway occlusion pressure: an important indicator for successful weaning in patients with chronic obstructive pulmonary disease. Am Rev Respir Dis 1987;135:107–113.
31. Montgomery AB, Holle RHO, Neagley SR, Pierson DJ, Schoene RB. Prediction of successful ventilator weaning using airway occlusion pressure and hypercapneic challenge. Chest 1987;91:496–499.

Chapter 11

Approaches to Mechanical Ventilation: Old and New

VARIATIONS OF CONVENTIONAL MECHANICAL VENTILATION

Assisted Ventilation

With controlled ventilation, cycling of the ventilator occurs automatically at a preset rate regardless of any respiratory effort made by the patient. With assisted ventilation (AV) the ventilator delivers a mechanical breath in direct response to a patient's inspiratory effort. The triggering mechanism is usually a small decrease in airway pressure as a spontaneous inspiration is begun (Fig. 11.1A).

As a means of ventilatory support AV was the first method to allow positive-pressure mechanical ventilation without the need to abolish a patient's spontaneous drive to breathe. Nevertheless, because of the need for a spontaneous breath, AV cannot be used to provide total ventilatory support. The safety of AV requires meticulous regulation of the triggering sensitivity. If the latter is too sensitive, excessive breaths will be delivered and respiratory alkalosis will result. If triggering sensitivity is excessive, undue inspiratory effort will be required and work of breathing will increase. Interestingly, Marini et al.[1] have demonstrated that this spontaneous inspiratory effort continues throughout the machine-delivered breaths and adds significantly to the work of breathing. The level of fixed ventilatory support provided by AV is often uncertain and difficult to adjust. Because of this, AV has been supplanted in many institutions by other options of partial ventilatory support, such as intermittent mandatory ventilation and pressure-support ventilation.

Intermittent Mandatory Ventilation

Intermittent mandatory ventilation (IMV) was originally used in infants with respiratory distress and allowed for greater patient comfort and better gas

184

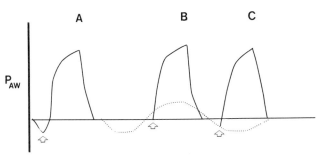

Figure 11.1.   Comparison of fluctuations in airway pressure (Paw) during spontaneous breathing (*dotted line*) with that during assisted ventilation (**A**), in which a small negative pressure triggers the positive-pressure breath (*solid line*). The same breath during intermittent mandatory ventilation (**B**) is delivered asynchronously, while during synchronized intermittent ventilation (**C**) the breath is delivered in response to spontaneous effort, much like in **A** with the "assisted" breath.

exchange and survival.[2] Subsequently, Downs and associates[3] provided evidence for the utility of IMV in adults in respiratory failure, particularly to aid in weaning from mechanical ventilation. With IMV the positive-pressure mechanical breaths are delivered at a fixed rate. These breaths are not usually synchronized to spontaneous breaths (Fig. 11.1**B**), which are allowed to occur unrestricted and unassisted between the cycled breaths. Because of the potential for "stacking" ventilator-delivered breaths onto spontaneous breaths, a synchronization scheme was devised. During such synchronized intermittent mandatory ventilation (SIMV), the mechanical breaths are actually triggered by the patient (Fig. 11.1**C**). If a time elapses during which the ventilator fails to sense spontaneous efforts, a nonsynchronized IMV breath is delivered according to the preset rate. Observations of patients suggest that such complexity associated with SIMV is unnecessary, since spontaneous breathing rates seem to synchronize with the ventilator-delivered breaths.[4]

Because mechanically delivered volumes are reasonably predictable, IMV enjoys great popularity as a standard technique for long-term ventilation as well as an aid to weaning. The inverse relationship between the patient's spontaneous contribution to ventilation and the relative amount of mechanical ventilation tends to maintain $Paco_2$ and pH near normal levels. The spontaneous breaths generated by the patient are not assisted in any fashion. Thus it is important with IMV circuits to avoid low flows and high flow resistances in the form of demand valves, lest the inspiratory work be increased excessively.[5]

Mandatory Minute Ventilation

Another technique introduced as a smooth transition to spontaneous ventilation is mandatory minute ventilation (MMV).[6] This allows the patient to breathe spontaneously from a reservoir or ventilator. If the minute volume during spontaneous respiration is less than a preset value, the excess fresh gas flow collects in a bellows reservoir. Once the preset volume in the bellows is reached, the ventilator is triggered and the volume is delivered mechanically. If, on the other hand, the patient's minute ventilation achieves the preset value the ventilator does not cycle. The MMV circuit also allows patients to increase minute ventilation above the selected value.

A number of benefits have been ascribed to MMV. Among these are better control of $Paco_2$, safety, and ability to provide a smooth transition from mechanical to spontaneous respiration. Like many of the unique benefits attributed to IMV more than a decade ago, these are unsubstantiated.

As a means of providing a constant level of ventilation MMV appears to have a major physiologic flaw. The typical response to fatigue or a declining ability to provide adequate spontaneous ventilation is an increase in respiratory rate and a decrease in tidal volume. This pattern of ventilation invariably results in an increased dead space ventilation. Thus a patient may move from apnea to tachypnea and meet the set MMV level while decreasing effective alveolar ventilation. The shallow tachypnea also promotes further alveolar collapse. Although some ventilators available for MMV incorporate low spontaneous volume (Ohmeda CPV-1) or high ventilation frequency (Engstrom Erica) alarms, the practicality of MMV at present has been seriously questioned.[6]

Inverse Ratio Ventilation

The technique of inverse ratio ventilation (IRV) involves the use of markedly increased inspiratory to expiratory time ratios (I:E > 1:1). The inspiratory time may be prolonged for as much as 80% of the respiratory cycle (i.e., I:E = 4:1). Inspiratory time may be prolonged by application of an end-inspiratory pause or by limitation of inspiratory pressure. The latter technique is referred to as pressure-control inverse ratio ventilation (PC-IRV). The peak pressure, respiratory rate, and inspiratory time are set on the ventilator and altogether result in a pressure type of ventilation rather than conventional volume ventilation (Fig. 11.2). This pressure limit is used to alter the flow pattern from a square wave to a rapidly decreasing exponential pattern. This is designed to allow "safe" initiation of a breath, since the latter is begun before expiratory flow from a prior breath reaches zero (Fig. 11.2**B**). Rather, inspiration begins when expiratory flow decreases to about 15% of its initial peak value.[7]

Proponents of PC-IRV postulate that the technique improves gas exchange by effectively recruiting alveoli and allowing better distribution of ventilation with the prolonged inspiratory time. With PC-IRV the benefits of reduced peak airway pressures compared to conventional mechanical volume ventilation have been touted.[8, 9] However, most clinical and experimental investigations demonstrate that the benefits from IRV are the result of elevations in mean airway pressure, largely because of auto PEEP or hyperinflation. Thus gas exchange and circulatory function are affected in similar fashion to other means of raising mean airway pressure (e.g., PEEP or CPAP). Further-

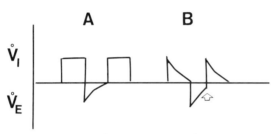

Figure 11.2. Flows during inspiration ($\dot{V}_I$) and expiration ($\dot{V}_E$) are plotted as a function of time during volume-controlled ventilation (**A**) and pressure-control inverse ratio ventilation (**B**). Note that $\dot{V}_I$ is a square wave in **A** compared to an exponentially decaying curve in **B**. Note also that in **B** $\dot{V}_I$ begins before $\dot{V}_E$ reaches zero.

more, the reduced expiratory time predisposes to air trapping and hyperinflation and the attendant danger of barotrauma. In fact, the incidence of barotrauma with PC-IRV is actually higher than that seen with conventional ventilation and PEEP.

Available data do indicate that PC-IRV improves gas exchange in patients with respiratory failure. However, the importance of the reversed I:E ratios or decelerating flow cannot be separated from the inevitable increase in mean airway pressure.[10] The enthusiasm for PC-IRV is tempered by its inherently uncomfortable nature, which requires paralysis and heavy sedation, both of which complicate and prolong the time until ventilatory support can be discontinued. Also, in contrast to volume ventilation, tidal volume and minute ventilation may vary widely during PC-IRV because it is a pressure type of ventilation. Thus, delivered volume is determined by the complex interrelationship between inspiratory time, inspiratory (driving) pressure, lung resistance and compliance, and the varying amounts of hyperinflation. Currently there are no scientific studies to support the use of PC-IRV, and the potential for misguided application of the technique is high.

Pressure Support Ventilation

Another mode of mechanical ventilatory support that has become available on many present critical care ventilators is pressure support ventilation (PSV). This mode of ventilation attempts to combine the elements of spontaneous respiration with a pressure assist that augments the patient's inspiratory efforts. Triggering of inspiration with PSV is similar to that with pressure-limited assisted ventilation (AV), but the termination of the inspiratory phase with AV usually occurs as soon as a pressure limit is reached. With PSV a plateau pressure is reached early in the inspiratory phase. Inspiration does not terminate when this preset pressure is reached but rather continues until the patient's inspiratory flow diminishes to about 25% of its peak value (Fig. 11.3). In other words, the preselected pressure is maintained constant by a variable flow from the ventilator as long as the patient maintains inspiratory effort. Only when the

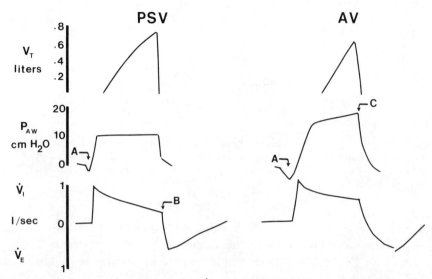

Figure 11.3.   Airway pressure (Paw), flow ($\dot{V}$), and tidal volume (VT) are depicted for pressure support ventilation (PSV) and assisted ventilation (AV) that is pressure limited. Note that both are patient triggered (*A*). Inspiration is terminated with PSV by a reduction in flow to 25% of peak value (*B*), whereas with AV inspiration ceases when a pressure limit (*C*) is reached.

inspiratory demand for flow diminishes to 25% of the maximum does the inhalation cycle cease and allow passive exhalation.

The appropriate use of PSV as a standalone means of ventilatory support requires recognition that it is not a form of spontaneous breathing. Rather, by administering variable amounts of mechanical support, a patient's spontaneous ventilatory work can be reduced. Thus PSV allows patients with mechanical impairments to achieve a larger inspiratory volume at a given level of effort or to maintain an adequate tidal volume at a lesser level of effort.

The principal indications for PSV appear to be in patients with high inspiratory work of breathing, such as that imposed by endotracheal tubes or ventilator circuits and demand valves.[11] In such patients, during weaning from mechanical ventilation the amount of PSV can be regulated to prevent respiratory muscle fatigue[12] and optimize patient comfort. High levels of PSV (i.e., those producing a VT of 10 to 15 ml/kg) can provide gas exchange comparable to conventional volume ventilation,[13] provided ventilatory drive is intact. The latter is important because PSV represents a form of assisted ventilation. The likelihood of hyperinflation and barotrauma with high-level PSV do not appear to differ from volume-assisted ventilation because mean airway pressures required for adequate gas exchange with both techniques are similar.[13] Thus, whatever benefits can be ascribed to PSV apply primarily to its use in weaning from mechanical ventilatory support where comfort and compensation for inspiratory work are important.

Airway Pressure Release Ventilation

One of the newest techniques for ventilatory support was introduced by Downs and Stock.[14] The technique does not involve delivery of positive-pressure breaths, but rather maintains airway pressure above ambient pressure with continuous positive airway pressure (CPAP) while the patient breathes spontaneously. The changes in lung volume that augment this ventilation are produced by intermittent release of the CPAP (Fig. 11.4). The pressure release allows lung volume to reduce as in normal exhalation, hence the designation airway pressure release ventilation (APRV).

The system for APRV includes a CPAP circuit that usually maintains the elevated pressure with a threshold resistor and high gas flows. At predesignated times a solenoid releases the pressure. The release valve must be of a very low-resistance type to provide adequate lung emptying. The volume released during each breath is a function of lung compliance, airway resistance, the pressure gradient above ambient levels, and the time during which pressure is released. When the valve closes, lung volume is again increased with rapid reestablishment of CPAP. Spontaneous breaths are possible at all times with CPAP or during pressure release. Weaning is thus accomplished by diminishing the number of releases until the patient breathes entirely with CPAP.

A feature that distinguishes APRV from other ventilatory support modes is the accomplishment of ventilation by decreasing lung inflation volume below the baseline maintained by CPAP. Since APRV applies and holds a set level of constant airway pressure before it is released abruptly, the pressure waveform has been likened to that of both pressure support (PSV) and pressure control inverse ratio ventilation (PC-IRV).[15] The dominant pressure with APRV is

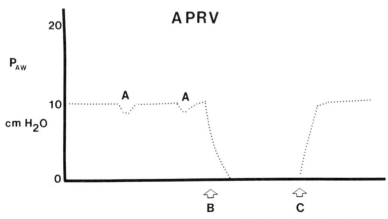

Figure 11.4. The *dotted line* depicts an airway pressure (P\ensuremath{_{AW}}) tracing during airway pressure release ventilation (APRV). The patient breathes spontaneously (*A*) with constant positive airway pressure (CPAP). Opening of a valve (*B*) results in release of Paw and allows an exhalation to occur. Closure of the valve (*C*) restores pressure and volume.

expiratory, while with the other two modalities inspiratory pressure dominates (Fig. 11.5). In addition, different factors are used with PC-IRV and PSV to initiate and terminate inspiration. However, the major difference with APRV is that the patient is allowed to breathe spontaneously at all times.

The clinical usefulness of APRV is currently limited by the lack of ventilators able to incorporate the rapid pressure-release mechanism. Proponents of APRV cite its lower peak airway pressures as a distinct advantage over conventional ventilation. Peak airway pressures with APRV tend to be about half those with conventional ventilation. Some of this difference relates to lung mechanics but also whether equivalent levels of mean airway pressure are reached. When mean airway pressures are similar, circulatory function and gas exchange do not appear to differ significantly with APRV or conventional positive-pressure ventilation.[14]

HIGH-FREQUENCY VENTILATION

Mechanical ventilation at frequencies more than 4 times the natural breathing rate has been referred to generically as high-frequency ventilation (HFV). Breathing frequencies with HFV are in excess of 60 per minute, and techniques encompass three basic modalities whose major differences lie in their range of frequencies. These are high-frequency positive-pressure ventilation (HFPPV), high-frequency jet ventilation (HFJV), and high-frequency oscillation (HFO). These techniques of HFV have received considerable attention during the past decade as alternative modes to conventional ventilation. Other

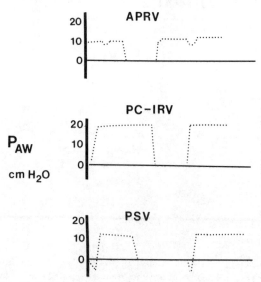

Figure 11.5. The airway pressure (Paw) waveform during airway pressure release ventilation (APRV) is compared to that with pressure-control inverse ratio ventilation (PC-IRV) and pressure support ventilation (PSV) to illustrate the similarities in waveform and the differences in timing.

nonconventional methods that use rates significantly lower than normal (usually respiratory rate zero) are mostly of historical interest.[16] This latter group includes apneic oxygenation, constant-flow ventilation, and tracheal insufflation. The tidal volumes and relative frequencies for these and the HFV techniques are summarized diagrammatically in Figure 11.6. The HFV techniques are characterized by their high rates and low tidal volumes.

High-Frequency Positive-Pressure Ventilation

The technique of high-frequency positive-pressure ventilation (HFPPV) uses much smaller tidal volumes (3 to 5 ml/kg) compared to conventional mechanical ventilation (10 ml/kg). These tidal volumes approximate the volume of the anatomic dead space (Fig. 11.6) and are usually delivered over a frequency range of 60 to 120 breaths per minute. The rationale was that such high frequencies and low volumes would be associated with decreased airway pressures and thus minimize barotrauma and adverse cardiovascular effects. Sjostrand and his colleagues[17] initially described HFPPV as a means of minimizing ventilator-induced blood pressure fluctuations in studies of baroreflex activity. They reduced tidal volumes and, to ensure adequate minute ventilation, increased respiratory rates above 60 per minute. Initially they used an insufflation catheter inside an endotracheal tube to deliver fresh gas at the high frequencies. Today HFPPV systems use a pneumatic valve system that delivers compressed gas through a sidearm.[18] This allows most of the gas to be delivered to the patient. An exhalation valve prevents entrainment of additional gases

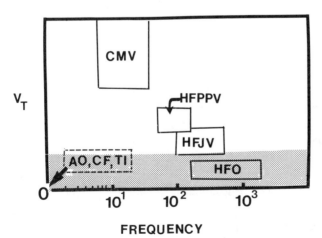

Figure 11.6.   Relative tidal volume (V$_T$) and respiratory frequencies (f) during conventional mechanical ventilation (CMV) and techniques of high-frequency ventilation, which include high-frequency positive-pressure ventilation (HFPPV), high-frequency jet ventilation (HFJV), and high-frequency oscillation (HFO). Techniques using zero frequency and V$_T$ include apneic oxygenation (AO), constant flow (CF), and tracheal insufflation (TI). The *shaded area* indicates the proportion of V$_T$ that approximates anatomic dead space.

and allows for application of positive end-expiratory pressure and better control of delivered volume.

Adequate ventilation and gas exchange with the low tidal volumes of HFPPV require that the circuit have a minimal compressible volume and compliance. This in fact is a prerequisite for all forms of HFV. The high gas flow in the presence of the low compressible volume produces a flow profile with a rapid upstroke to a peak value and then a brief inspiratory time (T_I). The T_I is usually only 22% of the total respiratory cycle duration (T_T), i.e., $T_I/T_T = 0.22$ or I:E is approximately 1:4.

Applications of HFPPV to the clinical setting have included patients receiving anesthesia for routine surgery,[19] thoracic surgery,[20] and endoscopic procedures.[21] Apart from these applications the clinical advantages of HFPPV over conventional ventilation in respiratory failure are unproven. Provided mean airway pressures and lung volumes are similar, oxygenation is comparable with either technique of ventilation.

High-Frequency Jet Ventilation

High-frequency jet ventilation (HFJV) consists of intermittent delivery of gas from a high-pressure source. The concept was originally applied by Sanders,[22] who used periodic jets of compressed gas to maintain gas exchange during bronchoscopy. With HFJV small volumes of gas (2 to 5 ml/kg) are introduced at frequencies of 100 to 200 breaths per minute into the patient's airways. The gas from a high-pressure (15 to 50 psi) source enters through a stiff, small-bore (approximately 16 gauge) catheter positioned in the middle or upper portion of an endotracheal tube. The flow is interrupted periodically by a cycling mechanism such as a fluidic or solenoid valve. As the high-velocity jet of gas enters the endotracheal tube, additional gas is entrained, usually from an ancillary circuit that can also be used to achieve humidification. This entrained gas adds to the jet flow through the catheter and results in a delivered tidal volume that exceeds the volume actually exiting the catheter.

Variables that can be regulated during HFJV include inspiratory time, inspiratory (driving) pressure, and frequency. Changes in these variables affect tidal volume and airway pressure and thus can influence gas exchange and hemodynamics. With most jet devices inspiratory time (T_I) is set at 20 to 30% of the total cycle time (T_T) such that $T_I/T_T = 0.20$ to 0.30. In terms of I:E ratios this represents settings from 1:4 to about 1:2. Decreases in I:E ratio or, more specifically, increases in T_I impair CO_2 elimination[23] and may result in gas trapping with stacking of lung volume and inadvertent PEEP. Inspiration is active but expiratory flow, as in other modes of ventilation, is passive and governed by the recoil of the respiratory system. Thus, as expiratory time is reduced by lengthened T_I, inadequate time for complete exhalation develops.

The inspiratory driving pressure is a determinant of flow, V_T, and CO_2 elimination. Increases in driving pressure over a range of 2 to 50 psi produce increased VT and thus better CO_2 excretion.[23] The high driving pressure produces a high inspiratory flow, which is reached early and maintained. This high inspiratory flow and further entrainment of gas are also associated with high mean airway pressure. The latter results in better gas exchange but at the expense of increased lung volume and greater hemodynamic effects.

As frequency increases from 100 to 600 breaths per minute, CO_2 elimination becomes less efficient.[23] This is attributable to the decreased tidal volume delivered through the jet and the amount entrained. Another consequence of the increased frequency is the increased gas trapping and hyperinflation. The latter explains why in most patients HFJV is most effective at rates between 100 and 150 per minute.

Clinical experience with HFJV has included its use in special procedures such as laryngoscopy, bronchoscopy, and tracheal surgery.[24-26] However, much early enthusiasm centered around the use of HFJV to provide ventilatory support in patients with bronchopleural fistulae. Massive air leaks in such patients often prevented conventional ventilation from achieving adequate gas exchange. At the relatively low frequencies common with mechanical ventilation the distribution of gas within the airways is a function of their regional resistance and the compliance of the lung parenchyma. With very high breathing frequencies, gas distribution is less dependent on the time constants related to regional resistance and compliance but more on the resistance-inertance properties of the airways. The presence of a bronchopleural fistula is analogous to a region of increased compliance, which during conventional ventilation receives a large portion of the delivered volume. With HFJV, however, the airway properties (resistance and inertance) dominate, and flow and volume no longer preferentially go to the highly compliant lung regions. On this basis HFJV has been suggested as a definitive treatment for patients requiring ventilation in the presence of broncopulmonary fistulae.[27] The efficacy of HFJV appears to be confined to patients with relatively normal lung compliance. In acute respiratory failure complicated by bronchopleural fistulae HFJV does not provide adequate gas exchange because of the requirements for increased mean airway pressures.[28] In the presence of noncompliant lungs the latter results in leak volumes comparable to conventional ventilation at the same mean airway pressure.

Other areas in which HFJV was believed to possess an advantage over conventional ventilation are its hemodynamic effects and effects on patients with elevated intracranial pressures. In both instances the advantages of HFJV have been ascribed to the lower peak airway pressures. However, studies have shown that the degree to which mean airway pressure is increased determines the amount of hemodynamic compromise[29] and elevation of intracranial pressure[30] more than the type of ventilation used.

In contrast to conventional ventilation, HFJV requires much higher flow rates to provide normocapnia. There is inherent danger in such high flow rates, which require high driving pressure. Any obstruction of outflow could result in abrupt increases in airway pressure and lung volume. Even under normal conditions, inadvertent gas trapping is a danger largely due to the normal expiratory flow limitation. The latter is particularly a problem in patients with compliant lungs with inadequate time for exhalation. Indeed, barotrauma is an ever-present danger with HFJV[31] or other techniques of jet ventilation[32] if adequate expiration is not ensured.

High-Frequency Oscillation

High-frequency oscillation (HFO) is a technique of ventilation that uses very high frequencies (up to 40 Hz) and very small delivered tidal volumes. Unlike with HFPPV and HFJV, the volume of gas is continually moved back and forth such that both inspiration and expiration are active phases. Lunkenheimer et al.,[33] in a correspondence, first described an HFO technique with small volumes delivered to dogs by a piston pump at frequencies up to 40 Hz. In the first applications to humans, Butler et al.[34] used high-frequency (15 Hz) sinusoidal oscillation and demonstrated improvement in shunt fraction and cardiac output compared to conventional ventilation.

With HFO, oscillations are generated by the reciprocating movements of a piston pump, loudspeaker diaphragm, or bellows at a frequency of 1 to 60 Hz (60 to 3600 cycles/min). The tidal volumes that result are well below the anatomic dead space (1 to 3 ml/kg). Because of the to and fro oscillation, HFO differs from other high-frequency modalities in that there is no net flow of gas from ventilator to patient. This is because the volume of gas delivered on the inward stroke is removed during the outward stroke. A continuous bias gas flow of desired O_2 is supplied near the end of the endotracheal tube to provide oxygenation and facilitate CO_2 removal. An expiratory port functions as a low-pass filter to vent excess gas flow (Fig. 11.7). The relationship between this exit port and the bias gas flow or fresh gas flow determines mean airway pressure. The latter, along with the inspired O_2, determines the adequacy of oxygen-

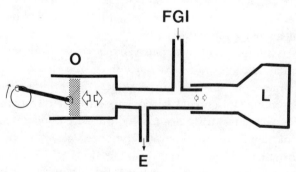

Figure 11.7.   Schematic diagram of a typical system for ventilation with high-frequency oscillation indicating bias flow or fresh gas inflow (FGI), piston oscillator (O), exit port (E) for gas outflow, and the patient end indicated by the lungs (L).

ation. Ventilation and CO_2 removal, on the other hand, are dependent on the stroke amplitude of the oscillator and on the frequency. Oscillators are capable of much higher frequencies than other ventilators, largely because of the active exhalation phase, which offsets the tendency for gas trapping even though I:E ratios with HFO are usually 1:1 and thus expiratory time is relatively shorter than with HFJV.[35]

Excellent CO_2 removal with HFO can be achieved despite the fact that tidal volumes are less than dead space volume. In fact, effective CO_2 elimination occurs with tidal volumes equal to about 20% of the dead space.[36] The exact mechanism for gas exchange under such conditions is uncertain but has been the subject of excellent reviews.[37, 38]

The principal mechanism for gas transport during conventional ventilation is bulk convection, which is also important with HFPPV and HFJV. With HFO, however, gas transport is more complex and convection plays a more limited role in comparison to other mechanisms. With conventional techniques, alveolar ventilation is determined largely by tidal volume (VT) and frequency (f). During HFJV the resulting arterial CO_2 tension ($Paco_2$) is inversely proportional to the product of f $\times$ VT (i.e., minute ventilation). At frequencies greater than 200/min, VT alone determines ventilation.[39] Increases in VT are produced by increasing driving pressure or cannula size, but changes in driving pressure are the most important determinants of CO_2 elimination with HFJV. Similarly with HFO, both f and VT determine CO_2 at frequencies less than 4 Hz (240/min), while frequency becomes a less important determinant at rates above this.[40] Elimination of CO_2 deteriorates above 15 Hz, presumably because of air trapping, elevated airway pressures, and impaired gas flow.[41]

The linearity of the CO_2 dissociation curve enables efficient CO_2 removal even if some alveoli are underventilated, because sufficient hyperventilation of remaining areas may maintain normocapnia. Adequate oxygenation, on the other hand, is not so easily accomplished. The sigmoid O_2 dissociation curve does not allow compensatory hyperventilation to offset ventilation-perfusion mismatch or shunt. The distribution of ventilation during HFO might be expected to differ from that of conventional ventilation in that it is more uniform and less dependent on regional lung compliance. Indeed, Brusasco et al.[42] have shown that, in HFO with a frequency of 15 Hz and VT less than two-thirds of dead space, ventilation was distributed uniformly between dependent and nondependent areas. The use of a frequency of 5 Hz and VT greater than two-thirds of dead space results in the normal pattern of gas distribution, i.e., greater ventilation of dependent areas.

In the face of a normal gravity-dependent distribution of pulmonary perfusion, a uniform distribution of ventilation between dependent and nondependent lung regions might be expected to worsen ventilation-perfusion mismatch. This does not appear to be the case, however, because of another phenomenon demonstrated during HFO, namely interregional mixing.[43] The real clinical problem with HFO and low $\dot{V}A/\dot{Q}$ or shunt areas lies in the inability of HFO to open alveoli and reverse the shunt such that other means must be employed to recruit lung volume, essentially by an increase in mean airway pressure. Thus, while HFO produces CO_2 elimination in a rather novel fashion, adequate oxygenation requires most of the same traditional methods for maintaining oxygenation as conventional mechanical ventilation. Recently, Walsh et al.[44] have demonstrated that periodic sustained inflations to 15 cm H_2O above mean airway pressure improved oxygenation and pulmonary mechanics during HFO. However, CO_2 removal was impaired in proportion to the increased oxygenation, much like what occurs with application of excess PEEP.

During HFO both animals[45] and humans[34] have been noted to develop apnea, some for long periods. This apnea occurs in the presence of normocapnia and appears to be a reflex inhibition of respiration. Thompson et al.[46] have shown that this is due to active vagal inhibition of central respiratory activity. In dogs, vagotomy reverses the apnea in spite of continued application of HFO.

It is well established that HFO can maintain adequate gas exchange in a variety of situations, including anesthetized volunteers[47] and patients.[48] During thoracic surgery HFO provided excellent conditions for peripheral lung work[49] but was unsatisfactory for mediastinal or major airway procedures because of marked changes in airway diameters. The latter results in loss of a large fraction of delivered volume because of airway distention. The authors felt that the advantages of HFO were outweighed by its disadvantages. These include difficulty in monitoring heart sounds and assessing the adequacy of ventilation as well as the requirements for high volumes of anesthetic gases. Furthermore, as with the other high-frequency techniques, expiratory flow limitation may be a problem, especially in patients with obstructive lung disease.

As yet there is no defined clinical role for HFO, yet the technique continues to interest investigators with its potential for treating pulmonary problems intractable to conventional techniques. This is especially true in cases of critically ill infants who are vulnerable to ventilator-induced barotrauma. Preliminary reports suggested that HFO significantly improved oxygenation in such patients.[50] Careful inspection of the data, however, indicated that mean airway pressures with HFO were significantly higher than those with positive-pressure ventilation. Thus the advantages of HFO were not adequately proved. What was interesting was the relative lack of adverse hemodynamic effects with HFO despite the higher mean airway pressures. Subsequently a multicenter trial comparing HFO to conventional ventilation in preterm infants indicated no significant improvement with HFO.[51] Rather the HFO group exercised a higher incidence of barotrauma and air leak. Thus the lack of objective advantage and potential adverse effects have led to the suggestion that HFO be used with caution and perhaps should be limited to "rescue" efforts in desperately ill babies who do not tolerate mechanical ventilation.

REFERENCES

1. Marini JJ, Capps JS, Culver BH. The inspiratory work of breathing during assisted mechanical ventilation. Chest 1985;87:612–618.
2. Kirby RR, Robison EF, Schulz J, Delemos R. A new pediatric volume ventilator. Anesth Analg 1971;50:533–537.
3. Downs JB, Perkins HM, Model JH. Intermittent mandatory ventilation. Arch Surg 1974;109:519–523.
4. Hasten RW, Downs JB, Heenen TJ. A comparison of synchronized and non synchronized intermittent mandatory ventilation. Respir Care 1980;25:554–557.
5. Meclinburgh JS, Latto IP, Al-Obaidi TAA, Swai EA, Mapleson WW. Excessive work of breathing during intermittent mandatory ventilation. Br J Anaesth 1986;58:1048–1058.
6. Perel A. Newer ventilation modes—temptations and pitfalls. Crit Care Med 1987;15:707–709.
7. Boysen PG, McGough E. Pressure-controlled and pressure support ventilation: flow patterns, inspiratory time and gas distribution. Respir Care 1988;33:126–143.
8. Gurevitch MJ, Vandyke J, Young ES, Jackso K. Improved oxygenation and lower peak airway pressure in severe adult respiratory distress syndrome. Treatment with inverse ratio ventilation. Chest 1986;89:211–213.
9. Tharratt RS, Allen RP, Albertson TE. Pressure controlled inverse ratio ventilation in severe adult respiratory failure. Chest 1988;94:755–762.
10. Berman LS, Downs JB, Van Eeden A, Delhagen D. Inspiration: expiration ratio. Is mean airway pressure the difference? Crit Care Med 1981;9:775–777.
11. Fiastro JF, Habib MP, Quan SF. Pressure support compensation for inspiratory work due to endotracheal tubes and demand continuous positive airway pressure. Chest 1988;93:499–505.
12. Brochard L, Harf A, Lorino H, Lemaire F. Inspiratory pressure support prevents diaphragmatic fatigue during weaning from mechanical ventilation. Am Rev Respir Dis 1989;139:513–521.
13. MacIntyre NR. Respiratory function during pressure support ventilation. Chest 1986;49:677–683.
14. Stock MC, Downs JB, Frolicher DA. Airway pressure release ventilation. Crit Care Med 1987;15:462–466.
15. Marini JJ, Crooke PS, Truwit JD. Determinants and limits of pressure preset ventilation: a mathematical model of pressure control. J Appl Physiol 1989;67:1081–1089.
16. Slutsky AS. Non conventional methods of ventilation. Am Rev Respir Dis 1988;138:175–183.
17. Sjostrand U. Review of the physiological rationale for and development of high frequency positive pressure ventilation. Acta Anaesthesiol Scand (suppl) 1971;43:1–43.
18. Sjostrand U. In what respect does high frequency positive pressure ventilation differ from conventional ventilation. Acta Anaesthesiol Scand (suppl) 1989;90:5–12.
19. Heijman K, Heijman L, Jonzon A, Sedin G, Sjostrand U. High frequency positive pressure ventilation during anesthesia and routine surgery in man. Acta Anaesthesiol Scand 1972;16:176–187.
20. Malina JR, Norstrom SG, Sjostrand U, Wattwil M. Clinical evaluation of high frequency positive pressure ventilation (HFPPV) in patients scheduled for open chest surgery. Anesth Analg 1981;60:324–330.
21. Borg U, Erickson I, Sjostrand U. A review based in its use during bronchoscopy and for laryngoscopy and micro-laryngeal surgery under general anesthesia. Anesth Analg 1980;59:594–603.
22. Sanders RD. Two ventilating attachments for bronchoscopes. Del State Med J 1967;39:170–175.
23. Rouby JJ, Simonneau G, Benhamou D, et al. Factors influencing pulmonary volumes and CO_2 elimination during high frequency jet ventilation. Anesthesiology 1985;63:473–482.
24. Flatau E, Lewinsohn G, Konochezky S, Lev A, Barzilay E. Mechanical ventilation in fiberoptic-bronchoscopy: comparison between high frequency positive pressure ventilation and normal frequency positive pressure ventilation. Crit Care Med 1982;10:733–735.

25. El-Baz N, El-Ganzouri A, Bottschalk W, Jensik R. One-lung high-frequency positive pressure ventilation for sleeve pneumonectomy; an alternative technique. Anesth Analg 1981;60:683–686.

26. El-Baz N, Holinger L, El-Ganzouri A, Gottschalk W, Ivankovich AD. High-frequency positive-pressure ventilation for tracheal reconstruction supported by tracheal T-tube. Anesth Analg 1982;61:796–800.

27. Carlon G, Ray C, Klain M, McCormick PM. High frequency positive pressure ventilation in management of a patient with broncho-pleural fistula. Anesthesiology 1980;53:160–162.

28. Bishop MJ, Benson MS, Sato P, Pierson DJ. Comparison of high frequency jet ventilation with mechanical ventilation with broncho-pleural fistula. Anesth Analg 1987;66:833–838.

29. Traverse JH, Korvenranta H, Adams EM, Goldthwait BA, Carol WA. Cardiovascular effects of high frequency oscillatory and jet ventilation. Chest 1989;96:1400–1404.

30. Shuptrine JR, Auffant RA, Gal TJ. Cerebral and cardiopulmonary responses to high frequency jet ventilation and conventional mechanical ventilation in a model of brain and lung injury. Anesth Analg 1984;63:1065–1070.

31. Egol A, Culpepper JA, Snyder JV. Barotrauma and hypotension resulting from jet ventilation in critically ill patients. Chest 1985;88:98–102.

32. Craft TM, Chambers PH, Ward ME, Goat VA. Two cases of barotrauma associated with transtracheal ventilation. Br J Anaesth 1990;64:524–527.

33. Lunkenheimer PP, Raffenbeul W, Keller H, Frank I, Dickhut HH, Fuhrman C. Application of transtracheal pressure oscillation as modification of "diffusion respiration." Br J Anaesth 1972;44:627.

34. Butler WJ, Bohn DJ, Bryan AC, Proese AB. Ventilation by high frequency oscillation in humans. Anesth Analg 1980;59:577–584.

35. Bancalari A, Gerhardt T, Bancalari E, et al. Gas trapping with high frequency ventilation: jet versus oscillatory ventilation. J Pediatr 1987;110:617–622.

36. Slutsky AS, Drazen JM, Ingram RH, et al. Effective pulmonary ventilation with small volume oscillation at high frequency. Science 1980;209:609–611.

37. Chang HK. Mechanisms of gas transport during ventilation by high frequency oscillation. J Appl Physiol 1984;56:553–563.

38. Slutsky AS, Drazen JM, Kamm RD. Alveolar ventilation at high frequencies using tidal volumes less than the anatomic dead space. In: Engel LA, Paiva M, Lenfant C, eds. Lung biology in health and disease. New York: Marcel Dekker, 1984: 137–176.

39. Benhamou D, Ecoffey C, Rouby JJ, Fuisciardi J, Wiars P. Impact of changes in operating pressure during high-frequency jet ventilation. Anesth Analg 1984;63:19–24.

40. Rossing TH, Slutsky AS, Lehr JL, Drinker PA, Kamm R, Drazen JM. Tidal volume and frequency dependence of carbon dioxide elimination by high-frequency ventilation. N Engl J Med 1981;305:1375–1379.

41. Hamilton PP, Onayemi A, Smyth JA, Gillan JE, Cutz E, Froese AB, Bryan AC. Comparison of conventional and high-frequency ventilation: oxygenation and lung pathology. J Appl Physiol 1983;55;131–138.

42. Brusasco V, Knopp TJ, Schmid ER, Rehder K. Ventilation-perfusion relationship during high-frequency ventilation. J Appl Physiol 1984;56:454–458.

43. Schmid ER, Knopp TJ, Rehder K. Intrapulmonary gas transport and perfusion during high frequency oscillation. J Appl Physiol 1982;52:1278–1287.

44. Walsh MC, Waldemar AC. Sustained inflation during HFOV improves pulmonary mechanics and oxygenation. J Appl Physiol 1988;65:368–372.

45. Bohn DJ, Miyasaka K, Marchak BE, Thompson WK, Froese AB, Bryan AC. Ventilation by high-frequency oscillation. J Appl Physiol 1980;48:710–716.

46. Thompson WK, Marchak BE, Bryan AC, Froese AB. Vagotomy reverses apnea induced by high frequency oscillatory ventilation. J Appl Physiol 1981;51:1484–1487.

47. Rehder K, Didier EP. Gas transport and pulmonary perfusion during high frequency ventilation in humans. J Appl Physiol 1984;57:1231–1237.

48. Crawford M, Rehder K. High frequency small volume ventilation in anesthetized man. Anesthesiology 1985;62:298–304.

49. Glenski JA, Crawford M, Rehder K. High frequency small volume ventilation during thoracic surgery. Anesthesiology 1986;64:211–214.

50. Marchak BE, Thompson WK, Dufy P. Treatments of RDS by high frequency oscillatory ventilation: a preliminary report. J Pediatr 1981;99:287–288.
51. HIFI Study Group. High frequency oscillatory ventilation compared with conventional mechanical ventilation in the treatment of respiratory failure in preterm infants. N Engl J Med 1989;320:88–93.

SECTION V

Appendices

Appendix A

SI Units in Respiratory Physiology

All science is based on measurements that require units in three primary dimensions of length, mass, and time. Most scientific nations adopted the CGS (centimeter-gram-second) system of measurement, which employed the centimeter for length, the gram for mass, and the second for time. Subsequently the meter was used as the primary unit of measure for length and the kilogram was used for mass to constitute the MKS (meter-kilogram-second) system. Other basic units such as the mole to indicate the amount of a substance were added to form the French "Système International d'Unités" (SI), a modern metric system.

The SI is a system of reporting numerical values that fosters exchange of information on an international as well as an interdisciplinary basis. The scheme consists of seven base units, only three of which relate to respiratory physiology (meter, kilogram, and second). A number of other units are derived from these basic units (Table A.1). Although many metric measurements in the SI system have been used widely in American medicine (units of mass and length), the use of SI units will require a considerable educational effort for physicians unfamiliar with their use.

As is evident from the terms in Table A.1, many of the derived units have their origins in names of famous past scientific figures. The SI system uses a series of prefixes before each unit to indicate decimal multiples (Table A.2). Otherwise, the use of each unit would make values either large and cumbersome or excessively small and unmanageable. The symbols for the prefixes are written before the actual SI unit without any space between (e.g., 2 kPa rather than 2 k Pa). The names of the derived units have largely been assigned to honor the great research pioneers in areas of science relevant to the term's usage. For example, when exploring the problem of surface tension in alveoli, the derived unit of force the newton (N) is used. This unit is equal to one kilogram-meter per second per second ($1 \text{ kg} \cdot \text{m} \cdot \text{s}^{-2}$). The actual calculation of surface tension is in newtons per meter (N/m). The use of N in the SI system supplants the term dyne in the CGS system. One newton is equal to 10^5 dynes, or

203

Table A.1.
Derived SI Units

Term	Unit	Symbol
Area	square meter	m^2
Volume	cubic meter	m^3
Force	newton	N
Pressure	pascal	Pa
Work	joule	J
Power	watt	W
Density	kilogram/cubic meter	$kg \cdot m^{-3}$
Frequency	hertz	Hz

a dyne is equal to 10^{-5} N. The unit of force (N) is further used to indicate the energy expended in various activities. Here the unit joule (J) replaces the term calorie (cal). For conversion, 1 cal = 4.28 J; 1 J = 0.24 cal. Essentially 1 joule equals 1 newton-meter (1 J = 1 N·m). This energy term (J) can be used to calculate performed work which, when related to time, is equal to power measured in watts (W). Essentially 1 watt = 1 joule/sec or 1 N·m/sec.

The general medical practitioner is most affected by the changeover from grams to moles, a basic SI unit not mentioned but designed to indicate the amount of a substance.[1] Respiratory measurements are most affected by the change in units of pressure from millimeters of mercury (mm Hg) or centimeters of water (cm H_2O) to kilopascals, both for blood gas data and respiratory mechanics. This measurement of pressure has been somewhat frustrating to clinicians because of the comfort and familiarity provided by the millimeter of mercury, which is not an SI unit.

Another unit, the torr, approximates 1 mm Hg or ¹⁄₇₆₀ of a total atmosphere and is named in honor of Evangelista Torricelli, an Italian physicist. Likewise, torr is not an SI unit, since in the SI system pressure is defined as force per unit area. Thus force in SI terms is newtons per square meter (N/m²), which is

Table A.2.
Prefixes for Multiples of SI Units

Scientific Notation	Prefix	Symbol
10^{-12}	pico-	p
10^{-9}	nano-	n
10^{-6}	micro-	μ
10^{-2}	milli-	m
10^{-1}	deci-	d
10^{1}	deka-	da
10^{2}	hecto-	h
10^{3}	kilo-	k
10^{6}	mega-	M

Table A.3.
Conversion Table for Units of
Pressure

cm H_2O	mm Hg	kPa
1	0.736	0.098
1.36	1	0.133
1033[a]	760[a]	101.32[a]

[a] Atmospheric pressure.

assigned the term pascal (Pa) in honor of another great scientist, Blaise Pascal. Essentially 1 Pa = 1 N/m². This converts somewhat awkwardly from millimeters of mercury, such that 1 mm Hg = 133.3 Pa or 0.133 kPa. Conversely, 1 kPa = 7.5 mm Hg or 10.2 cm H_2O (Table A.3). For example, an adult blood pressure value of 150/90 in mm Hg would translate in the SI system (kPa) to 20/12 (Fig. A.1). Standard barometric pressure at sea level (760 mm Hg) would be 101.2 kPa or roughly 100 kPa.

In the SI system the conventional unit of volume is the cubic meter (m³). However, in respiratory physiology the more traditional metric unit, the liter (1), has been retained to quantitate volume and flow.[2, 3] The cubic meter is one thousand times as large as a liter such that 1 liter = 10^{-3}m³. The liter is actually a cubic decimeter (dm³) or $(10^{-1}$m$)^3$.

PRESSURE

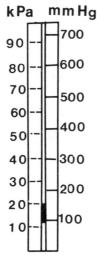

Figure A.1. Nomogram illustrating the conversion from millimeters of mercury to kilopascals (kPa), as might be used for measurement of blood gas tensions or pressures such as blood pressure.

Table A.4.
SI Units in Respiratory Physiology

Quantity	Common Unit (*a*)	SI Unit (*b*)	Conversion Factor (*f*)*a
Force	dyne	newton (N)	10^{-5}
Pressure	cm H_2O	kilopascal (kPa)	0.098
Work energy	calorie	joule (J)	4.18
Power	kg·m/min	watt (W)	0.162
Volume	liter	liter	1
Flow	liter/sec	$l·s^{-1}$	1
Compliance	liters/cm H_2O	$l·kPa^{-1}$	10.2
Resistance	cm H_2O/liter/sec	$kPa·l^{-1}·s$	10.2
CO_2 response slope	liter/min/mm Hg	$l·min^{-1}·kPa^{-1}$	7.5
O_2 consumption	ml/min	$mmol·min^{-1}$	22.4^{-1}

*b = a × f; thus f converts from common units to SI units.

The shift to SI units in the United States is still under way and is progressing slowly. It is led by many medical journals that require at least reporting SI units along with conventional units. Whether in the future SI units will become the exclusive common language of science remains to be seen. Table A.4 is provided as a background and guideline to the physical quantities that are relevant to respiratory physiology and the practice of anesthesiology.

REFERENCES

1. Young DS. SI units for clinical laboratory data, style specifications and conversion tables. Ann Intern Med 1987;106:113–129.
2. Hill DW. The application of SI units to anaesthesia. Br J Anaesth 1969;41:1053–1057.
3. Cotes JE. SI units in respiratory medicine. Am Rev Respir Dis 1975;112:753–755.

Respiratory Symbols

PRIMARY SYMBOLS

V	volume
F	fractional concentration in dry gas
P	pressure or partial pressure
Q	volume of blood
R	respiratory exchange ratio
C	blood concentration of gas
$\overline{X}$	dash over symbol indicates a mean value
$\dot{X}$	dot over symbol indicates a time derivative
$\dot{V}$	volume of gas per unit time (i.e., flow)
$\dot{Q}$	volume of blood per unit time

SECONDARY SYMBOLS

A	alveolar
D	dead space
E	expired
I	inspired
L	lung
T	tidal
B	barometric
a	arterial
v	venous
c	capillary
c′	end-capillary
$\overline{v}$	mixed venous

GAS PHASE

F_{IO_2}	fractional concentration of O_2 in inspired gas
F_{ICO_2}	fractional concentration of CO_2 in inspired gas
F_{ECO_2}	fractional concentration of expired CO_2
P_{IO_2}	partial pressure of inspired O_2

P_{AO_2} partial pressure of alveolar O_2
P_{ACO_2} partial pressure of alveolar CO_2
P_B barometric pressure (total atmospheric)

BLOOD PHASE

Pa_{O_2} arterial O_2 tension (partial pressure)
AaD_{O_2} alveolar-arterial oxygen difference
Pa_{CO_2} arterial CO_2 tension (partial pressure)
$P\bar{v}_{O_2}$ mixed venous O_2 tension
Ca_{O_2} arterial O_2 concentration (content)
$C\bar{v}_{O_2}$ mixed venous O_2 concentration
Ca-$C\bar{v}_{O_2}$ arterial-venous content difference

VENTILATION MEASUREMENTS

$\dot{V}_A$ alveolar ventilation per minute (BTPS)
$\dot{V}_I$ inspired volume per minute (BTPS)
$\dot{V}_E$ expired volume per minute, i.e., "minute ventilation" (BTPS)
$\dot{V}_D$ dead space ventilation per minute (BTPS)
V_T tidal volume (BTPS)
f   respiratory frequency (rate)
$\dot{V}_{O_2}$ oxygen consumption per minute (STPD)
$\dot{V}_{CO_2}$ CO_2 production per minute (STPD)
BTPS   body conditions, i.e., body temperature, ambient pressure, saturated with H_2O vapor
STPD   standard conditions, i.e., 0°C, 760 mm Hg, and dry (no H_2O vapor pressure)

SPIROMETRIC SYMBOLS

Lung Volume

V_T tidal volume
IRV   inspiratory reserve volume
ERV   expiratory reserve volume
RV   residual volume

Lung Capacities

FRC   functional residual capacity
TLC   total lung capacity
IC   inspiratory capacity (V_T + IRV)

Dynamic Flow Rates

FVC   forced expired volume
FEV_1 forced expired volume in 1 sec
FEV_1/FVC percentage of FVC expired in 1 sec
$FEF_{25-75\%}$ forced expired flow rate from 25 to 75% of forced expired volume

PEFR   peak expiratory flow rate (highest value for expiratory flow)
MVV   maximum voluntary ventilation

BREATHING MECHANICS
Pressure Symbols

Paw   pressure at any point within the airways
Pm   pressure at the mouth (airway opening)
Ppl   pleural pressure
Pes   esophageal pressure (used to measure Ppl)
P_A alveolar pressure
Pbs   body surface (atmospheric) pressure
P_L transpulmonary pressure (P_A — Ppl)

Pressure-Volume Symbols

C   general symbol for compliance, i.e., volume change per unit of applied pressure; for the entire respiratory system this is computed from P_A — Pbs
C_L lung compliance; computed from transpulmonary pressure (P_L)
Ccw   chest wall compliance, computed from transthoracic pressure (Ppl — Pbs)
Cst   static compliance as determined during period of zero airflow
Cdyn   dynamic compliance; volume change related to applied pressure at end inspiration during uninterrupted breathing
E   elastance, the reciprocal of compliance

Pressure-Flow Symbols

R   frictional resistance to airflow; ratio of pressure difference to flow
Raw   airway resistance calculated from pressure difference at the airway opening (Pm) and alveolar pressure (P_A)
R_L pulmonary resistance calculated by the ratio of transpulmonary pressure (P_L) to airflow
Rti   viscous resistance of lung tissues, calculated as the difference between R_L and Raw
Gaw   airway conductance; reciprocal of Raw
sGaw   specific conductance; Gaw divided by lung volume (usually FRC)

Index

Page numbers in *italics* denote figures;
those followed by the letter t denote tables.

211